# How to Master Stress in a Weekend

**MASSIVE ACTION**

**FOR**

**STRESS MANAGEMENT**

**ANXIETY &**

**STRESS RELIEF**

by

## Rick Smith

HPD, DHyp

# Preface

There are plenty of books about Stress, so why would the world need another one, and what makes this one different?

Maybe you are dealing with Stress or Anxiety for the first time, or maybe you've suffered for ages, and nothing else worked. Whatever the case, you're looking for results, otherwise you'll probably waste a lot of time and come away disappointed and disillusioned. You need a System.

In this book, you will learn;

- Why Stress is so dangerous to your health and well-being, and why you must attack it head-on if you are to restore some kind of balance and happiness in your life.
- What are the 'conventional' approaches to Stress Management and Anxiety Relief, and why many of them simply don't work.
- The awesome power of Self-Hypnosis, and how you can easily train yourself in just one weekend, so that you have a Secret Weapon to use, anytime and anywhere that stress attacks.
- How to take Massive Action to lift yourself out of inappropriate work or relationship situations which are driving your deadly, chronic stress.

Many stress and anxiety books nibble away at the symptoms without drilling down to the root causes. That's not what this book is about. There's nothing 'gentle' or 'new-age' about my approach. This book gives you the brutal truth about what stress is doing to you, and a decisive and effective battle-plan to combat it.

No-one is born to be unhappy, so do something about it!

## About the Author

Rick Smith qualified as a certified Clinical Hypnotherapist in 2006, and holds the NCH Hypnotherapist Practitioner Diploma from the Surrey Institute of Clinical Hypnotherapy. He regularly works with private clients around the world and also utilizes Applied Hypnosis and Neuro-Linguistic Programming techniques in commerce and industry, particularly in the areas of Management Training and Executive Development. In addition to his commercial consultancy, Rick writes and publishes on a variety of subjects, and now divides his time between London and Johannesburg, wherever the sun shines brightest!

## Disclaimer

I am not a medical practitioner and I do not claim unique knowledge or intend to offer medical advice on anything mentioned in this book. Any actions you take are entirely at your own risk, and it is your responsibility to consult your Doctor or a Qualified Medical Practitioner before making changes to your lifestyle which may affect your health.

# How to Use This Book

Whilst planning this book, I decided to check out the competition. After downloading some of the best-selling Stress, Stress Management, and Anxiety Relief titles onto my Kindle, what struck me was the 'light touch' approach that many of them promote. If you want to see for yourself, try clicking on the 'Look Inside' feature that Amazon provides whilst you're browsing for a book to buy (maybe that's how you're reading this).

If you're going to attack Stress head-on - which is our objective - then spending hours digesting the psychology and personal opinions of the author, and fiddling around the edges of your symptoms, is probably counter-productive. I think you want a solid strategy to completely eliminate stress from your life. So that is what I've tried to give you in this book.

At the core of this approach is Self-Hypnosis. Once we've examined the cause and effect of Stress and Anxiety, and the various established 'antidotes', some of which work, and some which simply don't (or are too complicated to be learned from a book), in Section 3 we're going to dive straight in and get you working on learning Self-Hypnosis itself. You'll have free access to four powerful recorded scripts, which you can stream or download, and which will train you in the key techniques, so that you can drop quickly and easily into hypnosis at will, and head off the rising tide of stress and anxiety.

I highly recommend you use your Smart Phone, MP3 Player, or Tablet Computer as the quickest and most convenient method. You can carry the recorded scripts with you, and you can use them anywhere, anytime. I have included instructions about how to do this on Apple and Android devices, and I'm sure if you are a Windows-Phone, Sony, or Blackberry user, you will be able to adapt these instructions for your own device. If you don't use a portable device, you can play the recordings from your PC or Mac, and even 'burn' them to a CD if that's the way you listen. There is no additional cost for this, and there never will be.

I've provided an interactive Table of Contents (e-book only) so that you can jump around inside the book, if that's the way you like to do things. Alternately, and I recommend this, you can follow the book in Chapter order, which will rapidly educate you in the realities of your condition, and then let you personalize and develop your strategies according to your own requirements.

Everything you need to know, and everything you need to do, is laid out in sequence. All you have to do to succeed is to follow the System.

If you enjoy the book and you find it useful, please take a moment to post a Review on Amazon. To encourage you to do this, I will donate the cover price for every review which includes the word trance (so I can recognize you as a genuine reader) in it. I generally make a charity donation for all my books, and the destination charity for this book is MENCAP, which is a British charity devoted to helping people with Learning Disabilities.

# Introduction

This is predominately a book for men, and the women who have to live with us. The stress that affects men is often caused by the traditionally "male experience", involving breadwinner responsibility, animal-pack job issues, and family obligations. Of course women encounter the same stresses in their work and relationships, however it is hard-coded into the DNA of men since time immemorial. That said, the techniques described here are equally effective for women, though the 'brutal' approach of this particular book may not resonate with the more sensitive female psyche.

If you've got this far, you're either stressed, or living with someone who's stressed, right? And if you've invested in this book, you've decided to do something about it. Right again?

There's no miracle cure for stress, no matter what you may have heard. Sure, there are drugs, such as SSRI's and Beta Blockers, which work pretty well for some people, but they're not without risks and side-effects, including the 'numbing-out' which many users report. And we all know about booze and weed; temporary relief maybe, but a slippery slope leading to a bunch of other problems down the road. There are 'talking therapies' but they usually take ages to work; there's meditation, which takes ages to learn; and there are a whole host of 'alternative' therapies like EFT (aka 'tapping') which have some anecdotal success. And let's not forget the old standards like deep breathing, which you should be doing anyway!

Frankly, if you want to take Massive Action, which is what you really need to do to beat this monster, you have two choices;

1. Change your situation so the stress triggers are out of your life, and/or
2. Master a method of controlling and managing your stress, instead of allowing it control you.

This book will show you how to do both, and quickly. The information contained here is a Weekend Boot Camp which you can do for yourself, with all the tools and techniques you'll need to succeed.

When I wrote and published "How to Master Self-Hypnosis in a Weekend," it was because I couldn't find any books which actually trained people how to master the technique properly. There were plenty of books that explained the method, but none that contained the tools needed to do it yourself. So I developed such a course, and I offer it permanently free with that book.

That book has gone on to be an Amazon Best Seller. More than 75% of the people who buy it download the scripts, and more than 75% of those people go all the way through the course. The book has great reviews and sits at the top of every 'self-hypnosis' search on Amazon.

Recently I have received numerous e-mails asking if it would be possible to develop the same techniques to help with Stress, in more detail than the original book. That's why I decided to write this one.

This book is in four parts

1. What is Stress, how does it work, and why is it so deadly?
2. The Conventional Approaches, and why they so often fail.
3. Self-Hypnosis; Your Secret Weapon. This section contains the updated three-stage 'Master Self Hypnosis in a Weekend' training, plus powerful new 'fourth stage' material that is perfect for eliminating stress.
4. Massive Action; How to bring about the life-change you need, to banish chronic stress for good.

Although Self-Hypnosis is central to this book, it is not necessarily central to the action you decide to take. I personally believe it is the game-changer that many people turn to once they've tried everything else. I would urge you to try it.

# Section 1 - Stress Unravelled

We tend to label stress as a symptom of modern life. Everything happens so fast, and if you can't keep up with the play, you might feel like you could potentially lose everything.

Alongside the well-known stress factors that are ever-present just by virtue of how we live, there's a whole bunch of more subtle pressures and influences which can also cause or amplify your stress. Things like:

- Troublesome or inappropriate relationships
- Career crises
- Alcohol and Drugs (cause and/or effect)
- Problems for people you love
- Money worries
- Illness
- Fear & Phobia

Stress is essentially a heightened state of 'non-relaxation' which is generally viewed as a negative or harmful state. People who encounter stress can often become strangely addicted to it. If you are in a state of stress, which may engender feelings of anxiety or panic, you are generally focused on activity to find a solution to the stress itself, rather than an analysis of the underlying causes or triggers. So the stress state can provide a distraction which stops you thinking about the actual issues, and concentrates all your physical and mental resources on navigating the stress itself.

However, there is nothing good about stress. It's not simply a mental process, but a whole-body experience which is driven and sustained by chemical imbalance.

# The Stress Chemicals

## Adrenaline, Cortisol, Norepinephrine

The three key chemicals in the stress process are Adrenaline (Epinephrine), Cortisol, and Norepinephrine

All of these are produced by the adrenal gland, located adjacent to your kidneys, where it can fire rapid salvoes of stress directly into your bloodstream. Norepinephrine is also produced in parts of the brain, possibly as a back-up if the adrenal gland is malfunctioning, which can have a wide variety of causes.

Simply put, Adrenaline and Norepinephrine are responsible for short-term elevations in stress, as in the well-known fight-or-flight response, whereas Cortisol over-production is the end-result of a longer and more complex process, and is responsible for chronic stress situations.

Everyone's heard about 'fight or flight' when the body adjusts to a threatening situation by focusing its resources on the essential survival functions, such as sight and hearing, muscle reaction, and suppression of fear. That's usually adrenaline at work, and in small doses it can be quite beneficial. Energy bursts, pain suppression, and a host of other 'super-powers' can be temporarily effected by adrenaline, which is essentially triggered in real-time by stressful situations as they occur.

Cortisol is a steroid hormone and is one of the most important chemicals that the body produces. It too is manufactured in your adrenal gland, and is essential for balancing bodily systems such as blood pressure, glucose metabolism, insulin levels and inflammatory response. The release of cortisol into your bloodstream is part of your primordial response system.

## Why Stress is Killing You

Heightened stress over long periods will ultimately shorten your life-span. In ancient times the constant struggle for survival meant that cortisol and stress, whilst useful as a protection mechanism, did not mitigate for longevity. For our cave-dwelling ancestors this was not such a problem, because there were a million other things out there that would kill them before they hit thirty. But these days, since we have medical science to keep us going well into our seventies or eighties, the cortisol/stress response is intrusive and dangerous, because it has not properly evolved to suit modern life.

So, if cortisol and stress are essentially unavoidable, unless you are one of those fortunate people who can self-regulate, you need strategies to deal with stress in order to suppress the damage it can do to your body if it is allowed to remain unchecked, the condition known as Chronic Stress.

An excellent way to approach this is to sharpen your Relaxation Response, so that you can come off the stress plateau quickly, thereby reducing your cortisol levels to normal. If you don't pay attention to this, over time a surfeit of cortisol can contribute to some or all of the following debilitating and often irreversible physical ailments;

- Compromised immune system, lowering your resistance to disease and illness.
- Hypo-thyroidism.
- Blood sugar problems leading to hyperglycaemia and diabetes.
- Leaching bone density, leading to osteoarthritis.
- Elevated blood pressure, heightening stroke and cardiac injury risk.
- Increased fat retention, a component of the dangerous Metabolic Syndrome.

The good news is that you can, with practice, train your Relaxation Response to deal with stress. Self-Hypnosis is one of the key weapons in your armoury.

The Self-Hypnosis technique for stress-control is quite simple. It's based on taking control of your key functions, such as breathing, muscle tension and heart-rate. If you follow the guidance and instructions in this book, you will be able to master these techniques. Hypnotherapists use these techniques to train thousands of people just like you.

However, knowing how to do something, particularly in a super-distracted state such that stress engenders, is not the same as doing it. For this to work, you actually have to recognize the stress symptoms as they arise, and make a long-term commitment to using a 'standard' intervention each time.

In addition, there are some quick-fix practical steps you can take in your everyday life which will lower the risk of stress symptoms occurring, such as;

# Caffeine

Everyone knows that coffee is a powerful stimulant. It also has some beneficial health effects, and it's a really nice and sociable drink, so nobody's advocating that you give up coffee. However, if you are drinking more than two or three cups in the morning, you're probably going to be wired by lunchtime. If you drink it later in the day, you may suffer serious sleep problems. Everyone knows this.

In stress-susceptible people caffeine will lower the bar considerably, meaning that even relatively innocuous triggers can provoke anxiety and stress reactions. Stress accompanied by caffeine 'overdose' is really tricky to counteract with hypnosis or relaxation techniques, because instead of managing your internal body systems to reduce cortisol production, you are fighting against an artificial stimulant.

There are numerous studies which appear to show that Tea is a fantastic alternative to coffee. Black Tea, drunk often and every day, appears to have a positive effect on cortisol levels, and L-Theanine, a substance found in Green Tea, is claimed to have many remarkable powers, among them promoting increased Alpha Waves (relaxation) and decreased Beta Waves (anxiety) in the brain. Tea is also a great way to stay hydrated.

# Smoking

Despite what you may think about smoking as a relaxation aid, nicotine is a powerful stimulant. Luckily it is a short-term chemical, and disperses quickly. The reason people regard smoking as a relaxation aid is because the 'ritual' of smoking when you feel tense is a 'self-reward' action.

How you perceive smoking actually has a greater effect on your mentality than the chemical action of the smoking itself. But you can be sure that if you are in a state of chronic stress, the ritual of smoking will only relieve you for as long as it allows you to change your situation, such as stepping outside the building. The nicotine in cigarette smoke will actually work against you and prolong the underlying stress state.

It's arguable that those heavy smokers who claim that smoking actually helps them de-stress are actually perpetuating their own stress conditions, but have been doing it for so long that they actually believe their own propaganda. Of course, everyone knows you should quit smoking, because in the end it will probably shorten your life considerably. However, when you're attacking stress, the last thing you'll feel like doing is trying to quit smoking at the same time. In order to minimize the harm of cigarette smoking, you would be well-advised to consider switching to electronic cigarettes. You'll still be ingesting nicotine to satisfy your craving, but you won't be putting your health at substantial risk.

If you're interested in learning more about E-Cigs, I have published a book called 'E-Cig Revolution' which is available in Paperback and Kindle versions on Amazon.

# Alcohol Misuse

Whilst it's true that alcohol is essentially a depressant, the incumbent ritual and social effects of drinking can have a profound effect on general mental health, and particularly stress. While a cocktail or a beer after work might help you relax, in the long run it can contribute to feelings of depression and anxiety, making stress harder to deal with. This is because regular heavy drinking interferes with neurotransmitters in your brain that are needed for good mental health.

Drinking narrows your situational perception, so if you are prone to anxiety, and you notice something that could be interpreted as threatening in the environment, you'll tend to hone in on that and miss the other less threatening or neutral information which ordinarily would give you a balanced view of a situation. This is one of the reasons why fights break out in bars!

Please don't dismiss this science too readily; it's human nature to believe we're in control of our drinking habits (unless we're already on the 12-Step Program of course) but the truth is, many of us are in a perpetual state of denial when it comes to alcohol. You don't need to go on the wagon, but you do need to be aware that your alcohol consumption may be playing a part in the chronic nature of your stress, even if you think that it's helping you cope.

# Diet

Dietary imbalance can have a profound effect on your body and brains' ability to cope with stress. Although carbohydrate-rich diets are counter-intuitive to a generally healthy lifestyle, complex carbohydrates such as wholegrain breads and cereal have an effect on your serotonin levels, your 'happy chemicals'. The problem is that simple carbs, such as sugary drinks and snacks, also boost serotonin, so stressed-out people often turn to these quick-fixes when they're feeling anxious or low. This produces a 'boom and bust' effect, wherein you gain temporary relief from your stress symptoms, but soon return to the previous state, or even worse. The habitual cycle ultimately impacts on your fitness, weight, and energy levels, and if you are caught up in this never-ending sequence, your stress will usually worsen as your health deteriorates.

# Disconnect Yourself

Nobody can deny the huge convenience of mobile phones, particularly smart-phones, as valuable tools for everyday life. However, if you are constantly on-call, particularly to a demanding employer whilst at home, or a demanding family whilst at work, your stress and tension is always there in the background. Try to set a schedule when your work phone is switched off in the evening and at weekends. It may feel strange at first, but like anything else, you will adapt, and so will those people who expect you to be on call 24/7.

By paying attention to the way you treat yourself, under the general heading of 'Mindfulness', and particularly the aforementioned stimulants, you will already be taking positive steps to lower your body's response to stressful situations. It's easy to dismiss such advice as "I've heard it all before" but there's a reason why these things crop up time and time again in health advice; they're true!

# Section 2

# Stress Management and Stress Reduction Techniques

As I mentioned in the introduction to this book, most authors and advisors on stress focus on providing you with personal strategies and techniques to enable you to manage and reduce the way that you respond to stress situations. Although my approach is intended to be more brutal and decisive, as in attacking stress at its source, it's entirely possible that you can modify your response to stress situations both short and long term, if that suits your purposes.

Here is a summary of the well-known techniques that you can employ to lower psychological and chemical imbalances which occur when you are faced with a stressful situation.

## The Conventional Approaches

## Breathing Exercises

Probably the most commonly used, easiest, and most convenient quick-fix for stressful situations and anxiety attacks is the use of techniques variously referred to as Breathing Exercises, Deep Breathing, or Mindful Breathing. We'll deal with the notion of mindfulness in a later section, but its true that controlled deep and rhythmic breathing can be enormously useful in helping to head off stress and anxiety when it arises.

Most people use relatively poor breathing techniques in their everyday life. Unless they've been trained to breathe 'abdominally', that is to say using the diaphragm as the primary organ to drive the intake and exhalation of breath, their tendency is to 'chest breathe'. This kind of inefficient breathing actually mimics some of the symptoms of stress and anxiety, and if you mimic a symptom, you can indeed induce or worsen the condition itself.

Musicians, particularly singers and wind instrument players, are taught this diaphragmatic breathing technique early in their training. In essence, it comprises both rhythmic breathing and asynchronous inhalation/exhalation, that is to say that by utilising the diaphragm as a 'pump', they can take in vast quantities of fresh air quite rapidly, and then exhale it in a controlled way in order to sustain a note.

Sportsmen and women also train hard on breathing, as in their case it's important to harvest the maximum amount of oxygen from every lungful of air, in order to feed their muscles and circulation for optimum performance. There are as many breathing techniques as there are sports and musical instruments, which goes to the broad versatility of the body's ability to utilize breathing to change the physiological conditions within itself.

It's not new age, and it's not magic, but since you have no choice but to breathe, you might as well do it properly!

The first thing to address is your breathing technique. One of the best ways to do this is to lie on your back and find out how well you breathe, with respect to whether you are predominately a chest-breather or an abdominal-breather. The common test is to place one hand on your chest, covering your sternum, and the other on your belly, covering your belly button. Then breathe slowly and deeply and judge which hand rises and falls the farthest. If it's your 'belly-hand' then it may be that you're already pretty good at breathing with your diaphragm. If it's your chest-hand, then it sounds like a good idea for you to learn a different way.

The point about proper breathing is that once you are able to control the rhythm and depth of your breathing cycle, you will be able to activate and sustain your relaxation response much better in stressful situations. You will avoid the well-known anxiety symptom of hyper-ventilation, which simply accelerates the state of panic, and triggers more damaging chemical infusions into the brain and bloodstream.

There are numerous training techniques for diaphragmatic breathing, and one of the better ones can be found at:

**http://healthland.time.com/2012/10/08/6-breathing-exercises-to-relax-in-10-minutes-or-less/**.

Once you have the basics, you should practice at least daily, when you are not in a stressful situation, until you are confident that you have mastered a technique that works for you without too much drama or effort. Then try it out the next time you feel your tension rising.

Breathing technique will also be an integral part of the relaxation methodology that you'll be taught in the Self-Hypnosis section later in the book.

The most important thing for you to remember with breathing exercises, as with many of the relaxation techniques that you can use for temporary relief from stress and anxiety, is to remain 'mindful', that is to say that you remain conscious of what is actually happening within and without of your body, so that you can 'instruct' yourself to use the most appropriate technique for any given situation.

Breathing technique alone will not solve your stress issues, but it will definitely help you to cope at a tactical level. It is an essential component of the overall attack strategy you will learn as you read this book and try the different weapons for yourself. This one's free and easy, so I would urge you to start practising your rhythmic, abdominal breathing straight away.

Various visualisation techniques can be applied to deep, rhythmic breathing too. Later you will learn all about one of the best-kept secrets of the human condition, which is that your subconscious mind can actually replicate a full set of feelings, emotions, and physical reactions to an imaginary situation, if it believes your imagination. So start preparing for that now by using colors in your imagination when you breathe. Green (inhalation) and Blue (exhalation) seem to work pretty well for most people. One theory is that Green is the color of nature, so when you inhale 'green air' you are drinking in freshness and nature, and Blue is the 'calming color', so when you exhale blue air, you will naturally induce a level of calming into your situation. As an aside, in anger management, they sometimes use dark foreboding colors like black and brown, to symbolize the exhalation of toxic and poisonous thoughts and feelings.

This may all sound a little new-age tree-hugger, and as I said in the introduction, that is definitely not the approach I take to stress, either in my practice or in this book. However, if a technique works, irrespective of where it comes from, I see no harm in adopting or borrowing it, as long as its practical application doesn't require any shift in your situational mindset (in other words you don't become what you use).

That's all I have to say on the subject of breathing right now, but you would do well to introduce it to your regimen, as it will crop up later in various places and techniques.

## Meditation

Meditation practices have been in use for thousands of years. The origin of meditation appears to be spiritual, though it is arguable that the technique itself is simply a physiological exercise designed to reduce the distraction of external factors and promote internal focus. Most meditation theory centers on the calming effect which can work in two ways for a stress sufferer.

In the first place, by taking active steps to relax physical body systems, it naturally follows that the action of the stress chemicals (adrenaline, norepinephrine, and cortisol) can be better controlled. You will recall that in the explanation of the physiology of stress, the presence of these chemicals is where the damage occurs, and by training your body to quickly shut down the response mechanism which floods your system with these damaging substances, it necessarily follows that your feelings related to stress will reduce and become more controllable. Meditation clearly has a part to play in this regard and if you are able to master it, it is an excellent tool for both short-term and long-term stress management.

The problem with meditation is that it is difficult to train yourself. Anyone over 50 will recall the amusing anecdotes surrounding the Beatles and others of their generation who went off all over India and Tibet searching for enlightenment, in the form of meditation teachers (yogis) and often supplemented by industrial quantities of LSD and other hallucinogenic substances. The key here is that even highly artistic people with (let's face it) next to no social or professional responsibility in their lives still sought out experts and teachers to guide them in meditation. In my professional opinion, it is highly unlikely that you can teach yourself to be successful at meditation. Even studying under a master is a long and difficult process before you will be able to achieve the levels of Nirvana required to achieve seriously satisfactory results with self-induced meditation. Don't confuse meditation with deep thinking by the way, because although they may appear very similar, meditation techniques are highly specialized, and we are not born with them.

Notwithstanding, there is a huge raft of material out there dedicated to Guided Meditation, which is where instruction is used, usually in the form of a recorded soundtrack, to assist the meditation student in achieving the necessary state for focus and introspection. If your stress is of the type which cannot be easily avoided, and you choose to go down a stress-management or stress-control course of action, then guided meditation may well be something worth trying. I'm not a professional in this sphere and therefore I would recommend you to seek out a good book on the subject. My recommendation is "Meditation for Beginners" by Jack Kornfield, though there are many others to choose from. Kornfield's approach is non-sectarian, and comes with either CD or DVD scripts.

## Aromatherapy

Aromatherapy is highly regarded for its benefits in stress and anxiety relief. It is based on the use of essential plant and flower extracts to promote health and wellbeing. The oils can be utilized either in direct application (massaged into the skin) or by vaporizing or diffusing using a variety of devices. The olfactory senses are triggered by different combinations of oils to trigger the generation of endorphins (pleasure chemicals) in the brain.

Extracts of lavender, bergamot, jasmine and sandalwood are particularly recommended for stress and anxiety, and can be mixed in various combinations. As well as the undoubted beneficial effects of the oils themselves, the 'ritual' of preparing and using them is (notionally) an important component in the whole relaxation experience of aromatherapy. It's a big subject, but if this interests you, a good place to start is:

**http://www.naturaltherapypages.co.uk/article/ Aromatherapy_for_Stress_and_Anxiety**

# Massage

The theory behind massage is that when pressure is applied to your body's soft tissues, it expels harmful toxins and releases tensions from your muscles. Professional massage can have a significant positive effect on reducing the production of stress chemicals.

There are numerous different types of massage, including Reflexology, which concentrates on relieving the reflex points in your feet, and Shiatsu, normally associated with shoulder and neck massage, which stimulates the 'flushing' of the lymphatic system. As much of the physical condition associated with stress manifests itself in tense muscular disorder, it stands to reason that a relaxed body can have a hugely positive effect on your mental and emotional state, therefore massage is highly recommended, particularly for chronic stress. A good primer on the benefits of massage can be found at the Mayo Clinic website:

# Self-Hypnosis.

Whilst meditation is a tricky area, Self-Hypnosis is significantly simpler and can be learned and practiced very quickly. The physical and psychological effects of Self-Hypnosis a very similar to meditation, in as much as the process is designed to achieve a deep state of physical relaxation, and to eliminate mental distraction, therefore calming the mind and enabling you to focus on serious consideration, exploring the mind, or simply reorganizing your behaviour.

Self-Hypnosis is ideally suited to stress management, because once learned it can be used in various different forms and contexts. Of course, you can sit down in a quiet room in a reclining chair and descend into a relatively deep trance (once you are trained) which will enable you to effect quite ambitious change on your own behavioural systems, or go into a process of deep consideration of a problem or challenge which may elude serious exploration during a normal day.

It should be noted that Self-Hypnosis is not a substitute for practitioner hypnosis, which is a much more powerful set of tools which can be applied to long-standing problems such as phobias and behavioural issues. Self-Hypnosis is more about effecting small changes in yourself, and developing coping mechanisms which will help you to quickly gain control of your physiological symptoms when stress arises. Once you have mastered the key techniques of Self-Hypnosis, you will be equipped with a system which will allow you to descend into a controlled state of physical and mental relaxation at will, which is a great escape route from potentially stressful situations.

In the next part in this book there is a complete section devoted to mastering Self-Hypnosis, including access to external audio scripts which are designed to guide you in the key techniques and training in how to induce the hypnotic state in yourself. I recommend you set aside a day or two and try this out for yourself. The success rate is, in my experience, phenomenal.

## Yoga and Tai Chi

These ancient mystic and martial arts are well-known for their beneficial effect when used against stress. I will not go into detail about them here, because in my opinion they are best suited to people who are trying to organize their lives around unavoidable stress, such as hectic family lives. These are very effective techniques and disciplines but require a different approach to that which is taken in this book. Nevertheless there is a huge raft of information available online and off-line, and if you are fortunate enough to be able to allocate several hours per week on a regular basis, I recommend you explore these options.

# Exercise.

Exercise is, without doubt, a magic-bullet for stress sufferers. If you do no regular exercise whatsoever, your body is not operating properly. You have evolved as a physical creature, and vigorous and sustained exertion is and always has been an important component of your body's functionality. If you want a really simple example of this, ask yourself why you get fat when you eat and drink? Then ask yourself why people who exercise a lot seem to be able to eat and drink as much as they want! Exercise is an important component of balancing many aspects of your physiology and your mental health.

The paradox is that when you are seriously stressed, even if you are used to regular exercise, you find it more difficult to motivate yourself. Likewise, if your stress is of the overload variety, you may allow exercise to fall down your list of priorities. It's hard to reverse this way of thinking, but you must give it your best shot. Tell yourself this: going to the gym three times a week may be a bit of a pain in the ass, but you definitely won't feel any more stressed while you're working out than you do sitting at home and worrying about it!

Remarkably, there are millions of people out there who simply don't exercise because they don't want to! This kind of phobic approach to keeping yourself healthy has nothing to recommend it. There's nothing right about not exercising, no matter how much you may feel that you are correct. The plain truth is that people who are physically active suffer from significantly fewer stress symptoms than those who are not. Internal systems work better, chemicals are more balanced, self-image is improved, and general health simply gives you a more positive outlook on life.

The simplest form of exercise is simply to walk. Owning a dog, apart from the obvious and well known stress reduction benefits, also enables you, and in fact forces you, to walk on a regular basis. Otherwise your dog is going to end up as fat and lazy as you are! A reasonably energetic 15 min walk once or twice a day causes muscle fiber activity, which increases your metabolic rate and has hugely beneficial effects. Brisk walking also causes you to breathe more deeply, and being outdoors exposes you to sunlight (at least part of the year) which encourages the production of vitamin D3, an enormously important hormone, allied to responsible stress management throughout your whole body.

Beyond dog walking, cycling is a hugely beneficial way to exercise, because it also provides you with a cheap and effective means of transport! You don't have to be super-fit to ride a bike, just about anybody can do it. It may sound simplistic, but if you try cycling, you will find that your entire mind-set will change whilst you're on your bike, as the beneficial exercise chemicals and endorphins flood your body and overpower the stress chemicals, at least for a while. If you can overcome your fear of being crushed under the wheels of the bus, you may indeed find that exercise such as cycling enables you to clear your mind in almost the same way as meditation, which is great if you are in need of some clear thinking.

I won't mention organized sports here because if you are the type of person who likes to play team games, tennis or whatever, the chances are you're already doing it and there's nothing I can add to that.

However there are thousands of excellent gymnasiums all over the Western world which are totally equipped to help you practice any kind of exercise, guided or alone. Ten minutes on the rowing machine is a great way to organize your thoughts and plan your strategies, because frankly there isn't anything else for you to do. The other advantage of exercising in an organized gym is that you can listen to your favourite music, another fantastic stress buster.

Many people avoid the gym because they're either embarrassed about how they look, afraid of how unfit they will prove to be, or simply because of some kind of inverse snobbery. This is all bullshit. If you're out of shape, the gym is designed to fix you, and the people that work there are professionals whose job it is to improve you physically. If you waddle through the door of the gym with 100lbs of excess flab you'll be welcomed with open arms because everyone loves to see a dramatic result. Despite what you may think (if you've ever walked in to the gym in such a physical condition), most of the people in there (and yes, people in gyms do look at each other) will immediately respect you for having the balls to get off your fat ass do something about it! Furthermore, there is nowhere else on earth where a grown man can look at hot girls dressed in figure-hugging Lycra without getting slapped or arrested!

Whichever course you take, you must exercise, even if you don't suffer from stress. I'm sure you'd rather not spend the final third of your life in physical degradation, perhaps even unable to walk very far or climb stairs, simply because you ignored the need to keep your body regenerating and active in your youth and middle-age. Regular exercise, however you do it, will prolong your active life, so you must not ignore it.

It's NEVER too late to start exercising. Just Do It ®

## Herbal Remedies & Supplements

Quite frankly, the best-known herbal remedy for stress is probably marijuana! There's no doubt that for some people, smoking or ingesting this particular herb provides both a relaxant and an escape mechanism from the stresses of daily life. However, it is not recommended as a serious stress management strategy, as over time it is more likely to induce a state of paranoia or ill-feeling in many people.

So onto the more legitimate (unless you live in Holland, Colorado, or Washington State) herbal remedies;

There's an enormous amount of claim and counter-claim regarding the efficacy of herbal supplements for stress, and stress-related conditions. The biggest problem with searching online for good information is that it's often hard to tell the difference between good advice and commercial pitch.

Livescience.com    http://www.livescience.com/16975-herbal-supplements-stress-reduction.html    recently cited Thomas Lenz, an associate professor of pharmacy practice at Creighton University in Nebraska, who published this excellent summary in the American Journal of Lifestyle Medicine. I paraphrase;

**Lemon balm:** Several small studies have found that this supplement, which is part of the mint family, can improve mood and induce feelings of calmness. One study found that 1,600 milligrams of dried lemon balm was associated with an increase in calmness for up to six hours. Lemon balm also appears to be relatively safe.

**Kava:** This herbal supplement is derived from the root of the kava plant, which is native to the South Pacific. Several studies have concluded that kava does significantly lower anxiety. However, the supplement has also allegedly been implicated in cases of liver failure, so it cannot be recommended on health grounds. It should also be noted that Kava, which is consumed dissolved in water, tastes repugnant and reacts very badly with alcohol. The effect of consuming Kava is a mild but noticeable high (a kind of South Pacific party drug), so it's not really suitable as an ongoing stress reliever. However, if you want to try it, you can order it by mail from Hawaii via the internet. As the legality varies from country to country, I stop short of recommending it or directing you to a source.

**Valerian Root:** This herb has been historically used to treat anxiety and sleep disorders. One study found that the combination of valerian root with St. John's Wort was more effective than the medication Diazepam at reducing anxiety. Low doses of Valerian root are considered safe when taken for less than a month. However, high doses may cause changes in heart rhythm and blurred vision, according to the University of Maryland Medical Center. It is always recommended that use of powerful herbs such as this are checked by your medical professional first, because there are known interactions with some medicines.

**Passionflower:** Studies have shown that Passionflower lowers anxiety in mice, but only one study has been carried out in humans. That randomized, placebo-controlled study was done in 2001 in patients with general anxiety disorder, and found that 45 drops of liquid Passionflower daily was as effective in treating the disorder as the drug Oxazepam.

**St. John's Wort:** In one study of 40 patients with social anxiety disorder, taking St. John's Wort for two weeks seemed to slightly improve anxiety symptoms; however, the difference between the groups in the study may have been due to chance, and the study itself was poorly designed, according to Doctor Lenz.

Many herbal supplements are sedatives and should not be taken with other sedative drugs or alcohol.

Dr Lenz's review was published in the November/December 2013 issue of the American Journal of Lifestyle Medicine.

The best way to treat stress over the long term is to identify the root cause of it, and change your lifestyle to reduce it.

If you decide to try herbal supplements for stress, you should be aware that they can vary widely in their quality and content. For this reason, you should consult a medical practitioner or qualified nutritionist before taking them.

So, although you may choose to extract something positive from all that, it doesn't sound like there's a miracle cure lurking in the herb cabinet, does it? Sure, there are always people that swear by one or more of these remedies, but they're rare.

# Sleep.

A common symptom of chronic stress is sleep problems. And it's self-perpetuating because the more stressed you are the worse you sleep, and the less sleep you get the more stressed you become. So if you're suffering from any kind of sleep deprivation, interruption, or other sleep problems, you need to attack his head on. The clinician approach to sleep disorders goes more or less like this:

## Sleep Problems.

Sleep disorders are almost always associated with external factors – nobody simply 'can't sleep', therefore in any remedial approach, it's first important to run through a check-list to try to identify or eliminate potential causes.

Lots of people suffer from sleeplessness due to one of the following 'controllable' reasons;

- Cognitive over-activity or habits which are not conducive to good sleep. You may be spending the pre-sleep hours ruminating, worrying, working, or pre-planning, and have difficulty in 'switching-off' at bed-time. The same effect can be caused by something as innocent as reading or watching TV just before trying to sleep.
- Nervous anxiety or tension, which can have many underlying causes.

- Unconscious fears or conflicts which affect your ability to fall or remain asleep.

Alongside physical relaxation, boredom is the weapon of choice to clear the mind of conflicting thoughts and mental interruptions. The legendary 'counting sheep' technique is highly effective once a relaxed state is obtained, although you may prefer to use something a little more contemporary and a little less fatuous. The objective is to concentrate the mind on something surreal or imaginary, in order to block out interfering or distracting thoughts about real life.

The simple process of focusing on total relaxation is usually enough to deal with 'standard' sleeplessness, where there is no serious underlying stress or anxiety involved. However, as it is stress which we assume is causing the sleeplessness here, you need to approach it in a more focused way. There are a number of practical steps which is easy for you to take, which at the very least will improve your chances of getting better sleep, and may indeed fix the problem very quickly;

## Sleep Hygiene

Here are some important practical steps which you should take to remove and eliminate any external factors which may be contributing to your sleep problems. Many of these sound obvious or even silly, but they have been proven to work over many thousands of interventions, so do not dismiss them until you have tried them;

Only sleep (or have sex) in bed, in your bedroom. Don't do anything else in that room. Don't read in bed, don't watch TV or listen to the radio or music. The bedroom is only for sleeping, so that is all you should be doing in there. If you decide, once you are in your bedroom, that you want to do any of these things, you should immediately get up and go to another room.

If you are still awake half an hour after retiring, you should get up, go to another room, and do something useful for a short time. Many people find cleaning works for them. After a further thirty minutes, you should try to sleep again.

Is your bedroom chaotic? Sanitizing the environment is important. Remove any clutter, obstructions, or unrelated items. Tidy up if necessary. It's important that you regard your bedroom as a place of peace and good order, or it will have a derogatory effect on your state of relaxation.

If sounds are a problem, consider the use of airline ear-plugs. They don't work for everyone (some people are disturbed by the sound of their own breathing) but if you are a light sleeper and you have noisy neighbours, they will help you to remain undisturbed.

Only go to bed when you are tired. Never take naps during the daytime. Do not sleep anywhere else in the house (on the sofa for example).

Set your wake-up alarm for the same time every day, even the weekends. Routine is really important.

Warm milky drinks and small carbohydrate snacks, such as unsweetened biscuits, just before bed time can raise serotonin levels, which encourage deeper sleep. But avoid anything else, particularly sugary snacks.

Alcohol may seem like a good way to get to sleep, but it is a very bad way of staying asleep. There is no known benefit to any kind of alcohol dependency, so if you are serious about sorting out your sleep issues, and your stress, less is more.

A hot bath can help. By artificially raising your body temperature, you kick-start accelerated cooling afterwards. Cooling is an important component of falling asleep.

Darkness is very important. Your circadian rhythm, the internal clock which tells you when you should be sleeping, relies on Melatonin to keep good time. Your own natural Melatonin production is suppressed by light. As we age, we suffer from reduced melatonin production; consult your doctor who may prescribe melatonin supplementation, which is highly beneficial for your overall health, not just your sleep patterns. In many countries Melatonin is easily available over-the-counter. When using Melatonin supplementation, it's important to follow a schedule:

- Always take the Melatonin at the same time each night, that is around 15-30 minutes before you would normally expect to go to sleep.
- If you stay up late, don't take it, or you risk disrupting your circadian rhythm. In effect, you will give yourself Jet-Lag.

- Once you've taken the Melatonin, go to bed, and make sure the room is dark. Light, especially blue light such as that emitted by TV's or computer/tablet screens, will screw everything up for you.
- If you wake up groggy, simply reduce the dose next time. Most commercial Melatonin comes in 3mg tablets. If that's too much for you (especially if you are young) try breaking the tablet in half.

Setting up for sleep is like setting up to do meditation or self-hypnosis. If the environment isn't right, any issues will be magnified, and distractions will interfere with your regular sleep pattern.

If you use Self-Hypnosis to relax yourself, and you want a simple one-line suggestion to repeat to yourself once you are in trance, try something like: "I may descend into deep sleep soon or a little later, and good sleep is deeply refreshing for my body and mind". Remember to keep the wording positive, and use (incontrovertible) alternatives. You'll learn all about this in the next section.

## Sleeping with your Partner

Do you sleep with your partner, in the same bed or the same room? Let's think dispassionately about this.

Why?

Sleeping together is a habit that is perpetuated (in the main) by culture or a sense of obligation. You meet your partner, you commit to each other, you move in together (maybe you marry) and then you sleep in the same bed for the next few decades.

Now, that might work out fine for some people. Maybe your relationship simply grows in a positive direction, or plateaus, and you find yourself perfectly in tune with each other's' sleeping patterns. You go to bed together, you both sleep soundly, and you wake up at more or less the same time. You don't disturb each other (neither of you snores, for example). Bliss!

Additionally, you may be in a phase of your relationship where body contact, intimacy, and sex are important to both of you. Congratulations if that's you, and hopefully you can sustain the situation into old age.

But the reality is often very different.

People in couples will often be prepared to put up with each other's' irritating habits or idiosyncrasies for the sake of preserving respect and love in a relationship, and sometimes this means one or other partner compromising on sleep quality. You may not even be aware that this is happening, because the prospect of raising it as a point of discussion is often considered to be taboo.

Many couples eventually face up to the fact that they are suffering in this way, and seek an alternative sleeping arrangement. In America, where houses tend to have larger bedrooms, one common solution is to swap the 'marital bed' for two separate beds in the same room. In Europe, where houses tend to be smaller, this is often impractical.

Perhaps you are disturbing your partner's sleep patterns (or vice versa), for example you may like to stay up and watch the Late Show, but your partner likes to go off with a book and read in bed. Maybe you have been used to watching TV in bed before you go to sleep (not a very good idea for anyone experiencing sleep disruption) but your partner is just putting up with it.

One habit of people who are stressed about their work life is to stay up later in order to drag more value out of 'personal time' and put off the inevitable (waking up for work the next day). Maybe one or other of you is off sex, for one of a myriad of reasons. Maybe you toss and turn, snore, or talk or even walk in your sleep?

In the earlier section on Sleep Hygiene, we discussed the notion that your bedroom needs to be a place of peace and tranquility, uncluttered, and YOURS. If you are failing to achieve this state of hygiene because of the significant other in your life, you might consider setting up a separate room as your 'own' bedroom.

This can work miracles for people's relationships and their stress levels. Think about it this way; if you set-aside the artificial and cultural reasons why you are sharing a bed or a bedroom, is there a real, practical reason why you need to sleep with your partner?

If you can identify any of your sleep problems as residing in this unnatural arrangement, you might try moving into the spare room for a few nights. This may require a delicate discussion. If you suddenly up and move out of the marital bed, this may be viewed as some kind of 'desertion' or "you don't love me anymore". Don't give up; just tailor your approach, such as;

"Darling, I'm not sleeping well at the moment, and I'm conscious that I disturb you in the night. Whilst I sort myself out, would it be OK if I try sleeping in the guest room for a few nights?" If you meet too much resistance, don't make an issue if it. You will have planted a seed, and made your partner aware that it is an issue for you. It's quite likely that in a few days, he or she will raise the subject again and this time they may be more amenable to the experiment.

If there's a sex angle, you'll need to handle it carefully. Everyone's approach to sexual relations in a couples' situation is different. If you are with a partner who likes lots of intimacy after sex, then it's going to require some clever and sympathetic negotiation to get yourself out of one room and into the other. However, experience tends to suggest that many people want to be left alone after sex, and your suggestion might be very welcome. In matters of sex, many couples are repressed in the way they discuss the subject, so your approach will need to be smart. At all times, be gentle and reassuring.

Because once you get that room of your own, you regain an amount of freedom which may help you not only to improve the quality of your sleep, and reduce your stress, but may benefit your relationship in other ways too. In its most basic form, you may experience a sense of freedom which, even if it doesn't alleviate the cause of your stress, may at least make you more relaxed at night.

## Chapter Summary

All the ideas in this section are aimed at making small improvements to your physical and/or mental well-being. In terms of how this impacts on your overall stress levels, you'll only find out if you try some or all of them. You may be surprised at how effective relatively small changes in your lifestyle can be.

You can chip away at stress, and you may indeed find that you don't need to do very much differently in order to bring about a noticeable effect in the way you relax, and the way you are able to handle stressful situations. If any of these work for you, Congratulations! You're on your way to a longer, happier, and healthier life.

Next, we're going to step up the pace. It's time you experienced Hypnosis.

# Section 3

# Master Self Hypnosis in a Weekend.

"The situation may be outside your control, but your reaction to it is entirely within your control"

The technique you are about to learn for dealing quickly with stressful situations comes in two forms; firstly, a technique that you practice daily (or even more often) in order to instil a long-term suppression of the chronic stress symptoms. Secondly, a quick-fix you can use anywhere when you feel the stress rising. These two interventions work well together, sort of like a 'parent and child' set-up.

Like any self-administered 'therapy', this will only work if you make a solid commitment to sticking at it. Human nature being what it is, we expect instant results. But stress is a complicated thing, which has both physical and psychological components. It helps to name it; "Stress" is the enemy, and once you accept that it is the focus of your attention, you will be able to deal with it in an unambiguous way.

The commitment model has three stages;

• Understanding and acknowledging that you are susceptible to Stress.

- Acknowledging the dangers of Stress, to both your health and your happiness (and others around you)
- Activating a personal plan to combat Stress and eliminate it from your life.

Once this commitment is fixed in your mind, there's no turning back. Nothing good can come of holding onto stress in your life, so why would you want to keep it?

The more you use Self-Hypnosis, the more effective it will become, and you will become very aware of how well it works. Come to rely on it, even become addicted to it. Once you have mastered it, you will be amazed at how easy it is to remain calm even in the face of tremendously stressful situations.

Remember, the situation may be outside your control, but your reaction to it is entirely within your control. You will soon have a technique that you have taught yourself, which you can use anywhere, anytime, to accelerate your Relaxation Response. You will learn to deal with the onset of stress during its short-term Adrenaline stage, and that will interfere with the longer chain-reaction of the Cortisol stage, thereby negating the risk of Chronic Stress, the 'killer'.

This is a 'tactical intervention' for dealing with stress as it arises. As you become calmer, as a result of mastering situations which would previously have caused you panic or anxiety, you will begin to find that the world slows down, and that you have a better overall set of coping mechanisms. Alongside these techniques you will also be encouraged to consider ways to manage your life more strategically, such as reducing chaos and introducing structure. The better organized you can become, the less unexpected situations will arise for you, and you'll soon begin to see that much of the stress we all encounter in our daily lives is directly or indirectly of our own making.

# Learning Self-Hypnosis

Hypnosis is a massive weapon against stress, for two key reasons.

Firstly, in order to combat any personal issue, it's essential to be able find clarity. You must identify the various elements that are responsible for your stress, and then focus in on the remedial action that you are going to take to combat your condition. Hypnosis, done properly, enables you to eliminate outside distractions, and concentrate only on your target. Basic hypnotic trance gives you an empty space in which to work. The state is completely internalized, so you suddenly find yourself with the freedom to explore your own mind, and to face and analyze your issues and concerns.

For the purpose of this exercise, we will call this 'Relaxation Trance'. It is similar in many ways to meditation, however competent meditation is a much deeper state, and often requires years of coaching and practice to achieve effective results. If you have the time and the money to take yourself off to India for a few years, you can become an expert. But then again if that were possible, you probably wouldn't be stressed to begin with! In my humble opinion, meditation is unachievable for, and incompatible with, a typical stress-sufferer. Hypnosis, however, is not.

The second aspect to the use of self-hypnosis is to re-programme your brain to deal with stress in a different way, and hence teach your physiological systems to choke off the free-flowing stress chemicals before they have time to elevate your body systems. Although your fight-or-flight response is hard-coded in your DNA by ten thousand generations of mankind's struggle, it's a relatively simple task to reset the switches so that it doesn't activate as often, or as long. To do this, simple instructions are used to train your subconscious 'operating system' to so things in a different way. We'll call this 'Suggestion Trance'.

# How Hypnosis Works

It isn't really necessary for you to know how or why hypnosis works in order to experience it. However, if it will help you to be comfortable with the process, here comes the science!

The established theory for the function of hypnosis goes more or less like this;

Your mind, that is to say the most recognizable manifestation of brain functionality, works on two levels, the Conscious, and the Subconscious (sometimes called the Unconscious, but this is confusing, a bit like Crabbies Alcoholic Ginger Beer).

Your Conscious Mind is paying attention most of the time. It enables you to interpret things that are going on around you, and perform conscious tasks which require some level of concentration or focus. Your conscious mind also acts as a 'critical faculty' making assessments and judgments based on a combination of logic and experience about all the information you receive throughout the day. It examines and decides whether the inputs are honest, reliable, safe, or useful. Your conscious mind can be described as a filter, only permitting some things to penetrate your deeper brain, and outright rejecting (or at least triggering suspicion) when it encounters something which is not so clear. It's your 'Bullshit Filter'.

Your Subconscious Mind, on the other hand, is running largely on auto-pilot. Inside are stored all your learned behaviors and assumptions about a myriad of things which are considered to be factual. For example, your subconscious mind learns how to manage your walking, talking, eating and so on, from a very early age, so you do these complex things automatically. It also seems to be in control of your memory. Any learned behaviour is managed in the subconscious mind, such as driving a car, riding a bicycle, swimming, singing a song, or playing an instrument. Also (and this is important) your subconscious associates emotions with experiences. Your imagination is very strong in your subconscious mind, and your imagination can simulate almost any sensation that you are capable of experiencing in 'real-life'.

How does your subconscious acquire all this information? Well, much of it arrives via your conscious mind, from your key senses – Sight, Sound, Taste, Smell, and Touch. Based on its decision criteria, for example Safety, your conscious mind will either admit or block a new input, which determines whether it is allowed to enter the Subconscious Mind, which has no such critical faculty and effectively believes everything it sees and hears. Without the filtration of your conscious mind, your subconscious would simply accept everything at face value, the bullshit would arrive unfiltered, and you would never be able to make a decision about anything!

Hypnosis, when done correctly, temporarily weakens the influence of the conscious mind, or even turns it off altogether. This enables information and learned behaviour to pass directly into the subconscious without any filtration.

Before we examine the value of this, it's important to eliminate the key concern that anyone would have reading this for the first time, and that is the safety aspect. Hypnotists are always asked whether hypnosis can force people to do things against their will, and the answer is an emphatic "No". There is a fail-safe mechanism in everyone's subconscious mind which is there to protect you, and simply will not allow anything dangerous to be suggested from outside which could harm you or risk any aspect of your well-being. Although hypnosis enables direct communication with the subconscious, it's not a dumb-interface, and if the instructions or suggestions don't fit within the subconscious framework of what is right and acceptable, they will not be accepted.

Now, inside your subconscious mind are all the habits and behaviors that you have acquired over your life-time, alongside all your fears and phobias. As you might say, you are the sum of your experiences. The problem with humans is that, along the way, some of those important things may have been corrupted by experiences, particularly when we are young, and before our critical faculties are fully developed.

Take smoking for example; If you had never come across smoking in your life, and at the age of thirty someone described to you a burning piece of chemically impregnated biomass which tastes dreadful, irritates your throat and chest, makes you smell terrible, compromises your libido, costs a lot of money, and will most likely deprive you of up to ten years of useful life, you wouldn't think twice about rejecting it as pointless, just as most people would reject a heroine syringe. But a young, inexperienced mind doesn't hear these messages. A teenager hears (sees and feels) adventure, maturity, rebellion, camaraderie and a whole host of other triggers. They light a cigarette and the majority are immediately addicted for the rest of their lives.

On a deeper level, many major psychological issues which people experience in adult life can be traced back to events or circumstances in childhood. We are shaped by the way we are nurtured, and even quite insignificant events can have a profound effect on the way our subconscious conditions us to relate to the world later on. In recent years there has been a spotlight on abuse, and how terribly some people behave been affected by things that occurred decades earlier. Only now are we beginning to fully understand this subject, and develop the resources within society to assist these unfortunate people.

So, when hypnosis professionals deal with cases where learned behaviour needs to be modified in order to enable someone to correct the way they relate to that aspect of their life or the outside world, the ability to speak directly to that part of the mind, the subconscious part, where such behaviors are stored and managed, is dynamite. A skilled hypnotherapist is usually able to completely fix huge long-standing issues for clients, if not in one session usually within a matter of a few one-hour consultations.

The technique required to establish this direct communication link to the subconscious is called 'Hypnotic Induction'. When you work through the exercises in this section you will experience induction a number of times. The hypnotism community generally believes that around 99% of all humans are susceptible to hypnotic induction, and those that aren't are from such distorted niches that they do not really register as a statistic; the mentally impaired, the psychopaths and sociopaths, and so on.

You may of course have heard of someone who states quite categorically "I can't be hypnotized". Hypnotists love to have people like that in their reclining chairs, because invariably the subject either didn't commit to accepting hypnosis in the past (which can be overcome by a skilled practitioner) or alternately they always were quite susceptible but didn't 'feel' like they were in trance the last time.

This raises an interesting subject, because the hypnosis experience is so widely variable across the population. Some people just go out like a light, lose any awareness of their surroundings, and have no recollection afterwards. They would describe the hypnotic experience as 'sleep' or 'coma', and they are invariably marvellous subjects who respond completely to any suggestion or therapy that is performed on them. Others will say that they didn't feel anything at all, but the treatments seem to work just fine for those people too. In fact, one of the 'greats' of hypnosis-training dared to say that if a subject complains that he isn't going into trance, the best approach is for the hypnotist to persuade the subject to *pretend* to be hypnotized. Remarkably, the treatments appear to work equally well in this situation!

In recent years, the medical fraternity, usually society's Critical Faculty, has largely embraced hypnosis as a valid treatment for a wide variety of ailments. I suspect that if the large Pharmaceutical Companies could find a way to make money out of hypnotherapy so that it didn't threaten the profitability of drug therapies, we would see a surge in its application for everything from pain control and anesthesia to addiction treatment and chronic illness. These days, the National Health Service in the UK and many Medical Insurers across the world include hypnosis and hypnotherapy as a viable treatment option.

Anyway, that's enough from the soap-box! The fact is, hypnosis works. And soon you'll know this, once you've learned how to do it!

## Practitioner versus Self-Hypnosis

The most over-used phrase in the hypnosis 'industry' is, "All Hypnosis Is Self-Hypnosis". Almost every book on the subject opens up with that as a mantra. Whilst it may be technically true on some level, it really doesn't help very much. It would seem to be more valuable in the context of training yourself to understand the key differences between Practitioner Hypnosis and Self-Hypnosis, because they are significant.

Hypnosis is not the same as Hypnotherapy. Hypnotherapy is a hybrid term, which should be clear to you. It's therapy which is administered whilst the subject, client, or patient is in hypnosis. Many of the therapies which are employed in this situation are very similar to protocols used by psychiatrists, counsellors and Cognitive Behavioural Therapists (CBT). The advantage of these therapeutic interventions when used in a hypnosis environment is that they often work much more quickly, because they overcome patient resistance (remember the Critical Faculty). CBT (aka 'Talking Therapy') can take tens or even hundreds of hours to fix a phobia that a competent hypnotherapist can deal with in a couple of sessions.

Again, we'll use the smoking analogy. The success rate of hypnotherapy in smoking cessation is well-documented as being one of the very best methods of all, being statistically far more successful than Nicotine Replacement Therapy (NRT), Zyban or any of the Health Education initiatives. Probably the only thing that's worked better in the last ten years was banning smoking in pubs, until E-Cigs came along at least! Now if you were to read the hypnotherapist's Stop-Smoking 'script' to yourself, without hypnosis, it would sound bland and trite, and somewhat childish in places. You cannot imagine that reading, or being read, that monolog would have any effect on your smoking habit. However, when administered in the hypnosis environment by an experienced therapist, the results are simply staggering. A substantial percentage of clients stop smoking for more than six months, and many go on to live tobacco-free for their whole lives! Intriguingly, one of the key success factors for this treatment is that the client must PAY for the treatment. If you give it for free, success rates plummet.

So, to our comparison. I would safely say that using a conventional Stop-Smoking script in Self-Hypnosis will not achieve the success rate of that in the hands of a professional hypnotherapist. It's not only because of the financial aspect, but also a whole host of other 'human nature' issues which are too expansive to explore in this book. Practitioner hypnosis is useful when massive change is the objective.

Self-hypnosis is more subtle, but it also possesses some unique advantages. For a start, because it's free, and you can use it according to your own schedule, it's a much more convenient thing to repeat over and over again, and repetition is a key tool in the hypnosis toolbox.

Self-Hypnosis can be used very effectively to improve confidence, alleviate anxiety or performance pressure, strengthen commitment, and in all sorts of situations where the subject suffers from cognitive irrationality: that is that they know they are reacting inappropriately to a situation and are capable of focusing on fact, rather than succumbing to emotion. In the self-hypnotic trance state, the distracting triggers are suppressed, and the subject is able to zoom in on the correct way to behave, thereby strengthening the 'model' which can be used to get through a difficult or challenging situation. Whilst practitioner hypnosis is highly effective in these situations, it's clearly impossible to have a hypnotherapist alongside you all the time, so the ability to quickly drop into trance and perform a predetermined routine can be highly effective in providing a quick-fix.

Most people find it impossible to memorize long scripts and then carry them into the trance state so that they can use them for 'therapy', and any Self-Hypnosis training which suggests otherwise is probably going to be unsuccessful for most people. So, for Self-Hypnosis to be an effective tool for changing yourself, it's important to use strong but simple self-suggestions which are easy to memorize and execute once the induction has taken place.

For specifically targeted change, these suggestions should take the form of 'one-liners', which when used repetitively will lodge in the subconscious and become automatic calls to action whenever the particular situation occurs.

In the Bonus Material at the end of this book, we will examine some of these techniques further, and you'll learn how to write really effective mini-scripts which obey the golden rules of hypnotic suggestion.

But for now, let's get on and train you to do Self-Hypnosis, and then build from there.

# Preparation and Set-Up

In my original book "How to Master Self-Hypnosis in a Weekend' I offered readers the option to use my pre-recorded scripts, or alternately to record the scripts for themselves, using transcripts included in the book's text. From the feedback I have received, and also my tracking and monitoring of the script recordings online, I am fairly sure that nobody bothered recording them themselves, so I have not included any transcripts in this book. If, for some reason of your own, you would like to obtain the transcripts, you can e-mail me and I will send them to you. My contact information is listed at the end.

I will therefore assume that you have a device that can stream or download MP3 files from the internet, which is the optimum way to use the material. Of course, it's free, since you already paid for the book.

In this Chapter, we're going to look at two important practical aspects of Self-Hypnosis;

- How to access and use the Recorded Scripts, using your Computer, Smartphone or Tablet
- Preparing and setting up your Self-Hypnosis 'Zone'.


# How to Use the Scripts.

To gain access to the Recorded Exercises (the "Scripts") please click on this link, or type it into your Browser:

**http://tiny.cc/2f0eex**

Alternately you can type or copy it into your Web Browser. Once you click the link, you will be taken to a web page which will ask for your name and your e-mail address. Once you hit 'enter', you will receive an e-mail containing the direct links to the recordings themselves. Once you have these links, you are free to use the scripts as often as you like, on any device.

Just a note on data protection; under no circumstances will your e-mail address ever be shared. From time to time, I may e-mail you about updates and supplementary material, or new books I publish, but your data will never be used for any external purposes. Your confidentiality is completely assured.

Why not click through immediately, then you will be ready to start the exercises at your convenience.

The first script we are going to use is called 'Exercise One; Basic Induction and Emerge' and it can be found using the link. Don't click it just yet; it's repeated again later.

It's an MP3 file, which means it will play on just about any device, and it's around 15Mb, so it's really quite small. It lasts around 15 minutes.

## Stream to your Smartphone or iPod

If you are reading this on a smartphone or tablet, you should be able to complete the process, then click straight through and stream it in a couple of minutes (but please read the rest of this chapter before you begin!). Alternately if you copy or type the link you receive into your Smartphone's web browser, you can play the file directly from the web. This means you can access it from anywhere that you have data access, though I would recommend you don't use Contract Data with your Phone Carrier unless you have a large or unlimited data bundle. Wi-fi, particularly at home, is usually free, so that's the best and most reliable way to access the script. Whenever you use your phone for playing scripts, which you'll be doing a lot throughout this course, please use headphones for privacy. This also helps to block out external noises which can be a distraction during your Self-Hypnosis sessions.

Tablets, such as the iPad, Kindle Fire, Google Nexus and Microsoft Surface will allow you to play the file directly. Older Kindles do not have sound, so you'll need to use the link on another device.

## Download to your Computer

You can use your Computer's web browser, by copying or typing the link from the e-mail, and the audio file will open (it may start to play). I recommend you pause the audio, then right-click (Command-Click on a Mac) on it, selecting 'Save Audio As'. This should open a file saving dialog box, and you can download and save the MP3 file in your Music Library. Once you've done that, you can open your Music Player (such as iTunes) and find the track in the alphabetic list of all your stored music tracks. The artist name is Rick Smith.

These instructions are repeated in the e-mail you will receive with the links.

Alternately, if you download it to your 'Downloads' or 'Desktop', you can then open iTunes or your preferred Music Player, and import the file from there.

You can play it from there, or alternately you might decide to create a new Playlist (call it "Self Hypnosis") and drag the track into it. Then you will easily be able to find it, and when you sync to your device next time, make sure you add the playlist and you'll be able to find it easily on your phone or tablet, which is where you really need it to be.

Occasionally I am contacted by my readers complaining that they cannot access the scripts. I personally check the links and recordings on various devices every few days, to ensure that they are working properly (which they always are). So if you hit a snag, the likelihood is that you have a problem at your end! If this persists, please e-mail me on ricksmith@zonehypnosis.com and I will send you alternate 'emergency links' which by-pass the various stages where you may be experiencing difficulties. If you are attempting to access the scripts from your work IT network and you hit a problem, it may be because your organization's IT policy prevents access to the "tiny.cc" server that I use to track the link usage. I recently had a client mail me from a certain US Corrections facility, who was experiencing exactly this problem!

Once again, here's the link you need to get started:

**http://tiny.cc/2f0eex**

## Set-Up and Preparation

In order to give yourself the best opportunity for success with Self-Hypnosis, we need to pay attention to your immediate environment. The more ideal we can make the set-up, the more relaxed you will become and the fewer distractions are likely to occur. Most of these instructions are simple common sense, but you'd be surprised at how many people ignore the obvious!

## Privacy

In the early stages, whilst you're learning the basics, you need to shut yourself away somewhere private, and make sure you won't be disturbed. Self-Hypnosis is a solitary pastime; the clue is in the title: *SELF*-Hypnosis, and there's nothing to be gained by having someone else listening in or involving themselves in the process. If you live alone it's simple. If you have family, particularly a parent, sibling or partner, it's up to you if you decide to tell them what you are planning to do. However, it's always better to come clean, because when you finally shut yourself away to practice you really need to have eliminated any concerns that you are doing something covert or sneaky, or that someone might think of you as foolish or flippant if they accidentally discover what you are doing. Hypnosis always works better if you are free of short-term worries. You don't want to be trying to induce a trance whilst keeping one ear open for approaching footsteps! Whatever the case, they need to understand that whilst you are practicing Self-Hypnosis, they should not disturb you unless the house is burning down! As for kids: well I think you know the answer to that! But seriously, if you are going to eliminate distraction, which is necessary for this process to work, you must *control your environment.*

## Tranquillity

Silence in your hypnosis environment is ideal, though it may be impossible to achieve total peace and quiet, especially if you live in a city. Nevertheless you should strive to establish the quietest possible space for your Self-Hypnosis. Close the doors and windows and switch your phone to 'Flight Mode' so that it won't ring or vibrate. Anything which disrupts your concentration whilst you are doing the exercise will necessarily take you back to the beginning. Once you are well-practiced at this, you will be able to deal with external sounds as part of the trance, but at the beginning, until you have mastered the process, you need to eliminate as much external disturbance as possible.

Pets can be a particular problem, especially dogs. I once visited a client in her home, and I was quite concerned to find that she had an open plan house and four pet dogs, including two huge German Shepherd 'guard dogs' who barked like crazy when she tried to shut them outside. I decided that the lesser of two evils was to have the dogs in the room with us whilst we did the session. They spent the whole hour licking her, climbing on and off chairs, and generally making a nuisance of themselves. I had travelled a long way to see her and she was paying a lot for the therapy, so I was forced to improvise by incorporating the dogs into the hypnotic induction, so that she was able to ignore them. It took a little longer than usual to get her into a workable trance, but I stuck at it and the session was, in the end, completely successful. However, I am a professional and I know how to do these bizarre things from time to time. I doubt you will be able to manage anything like this when you are doing hypnosis alone, so don't try.

If there are sounds in the room, such as a ticking clock (preferably you should move it or stop it temporarily) an air-conditioning unit, or anything else, you need to take some time in your preparation to get used to the ambient sounds, because you may have never really listened to them before. The idea is that you merge all sounds into the background environment so that they do not become intrusive. Once you get your trance going, you will either not notice them at all, or alternately they may simply become part of the comforting aspects of your environment.

Remember, you should be using headphones to listen to the scripts in this first phase. If you are using ear-buds, external sounds will break through quite easily. However, if you can use a pair of over-ear or even noise-cancelling headphones, external sounds should not be a problem. I have often used headphones for my clients and a headset microphone for myself in my London practice, which is just 1800ft beneath the flight path for Heathrow airport!

## Your Personal Comforts

As you have understood, achieving the hypnotic trance state will always go better if you eliminate distractions, which includes physical distractions. Wear clothing that doesn't pinch or constrict (you may want to remove your shoes, belt, and wrist-watch, just like the last time you were locked up by the cops). Please make sure you visit the bathroom before you start, because although a full bladder may indeed focus the mind in business meetings, a call of nature half-way through your hypnosis session is difficult to ignore, and again it will probably require you to start the induction all over again. Make sure the room temperature is comfortable, not too cool and not too warm.

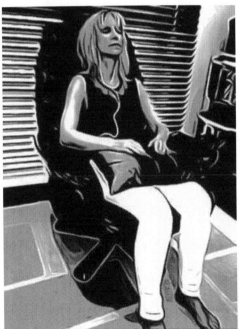

## Where to Sit

If you've ever visit a hypnotherapist, you will rarely see a couch or flat-bed in his or her office, and there's a good reason for this. As you can imagine, taking people into a state of deep relaxation can run the risk of them falling asleep, especially if they arrive tired for the session. If you are lying down the risk is increased, because this is most people's natural sleeping position. If a subject nods off during hypnosis, the session is essentially wasted, because the aural senses shut down as soon as you are asleep and nothing goes in, apart from the noise of a fire alarm or a wake-up call of course. Falling asleep during hypnosis is not uncommon, and it is completely harmless. Once asleep, the hypnosis is essentially over, and anything that happens whilst you are asleep won't be effective. But at least you'll have a nice little nap!

Within the scope of the hypnosis exercises you will do in this course, you can be sure that you will eventually wake up 'out of trance', so no harm done. But you could waste some time and effort, which is why you should try to avoid lying horizontally if possible. Of course, if you have no alternative comfortable location, the hypnosis itself will work fine on a couch or bed, but you need to be aware of the heightened risk of sleeping through the best bit!

The ideal situation is a comfortable chair: a recliner if you have access to one. A Lazy Boy is not ideal, unless you can lock out the leg-rest, because the very best seating position for hypnosis is to have your legs uncrossed and your feet flat on the floor. You should make sure your head and neck are supported if possible. If you have one of those horseshoe-shaped travel pillows, use it.

Where to put your hands is really related to how you would normally sit to relax. I have found that most clients like it if I give them cushion to put on their lap and then they can rest their hands on it. A competent professional hypnotist can work on clients in almost any position, and if you've ever seen a good stage hypnotist, you'll have seen subjects put into trance whilst standing up. This is genuine, but it takes training to master. For your purposes, you should try to get as close to the picture as you can manage. As long as you're comfortable, and you don't need to tense any muscles to maintain your position, this will work just fine.

## Stimulants

Stimulants can be an issue, so you should avoid them. Coffee in particular can inhibit relaxation, so it is best to avoid drinking it at all on the days you are going to work on your Self-Hypnosis skills. Later, once you have mastered dropping in and out of trance at will, it won't make much difference, but in the early stages you are trying to eliminate every possible obstacle to you being able to enjoy the relaxation state that leads to hypnotic trance.

If you are a smoker, I recommend that you thoroughly cleanse your breath and hands before you start. In hypnosis, senses can sometimes sharpen unexpectedly, and the smell of tobacco could become intrusive once all other distractions are suppressed or eliminated, which could trigger a craving.

Of course – and this probably goes without saying – alcohol and drugs don't go well with hypnosis. It's virtually impossible to hypnotize a drunk, although I did once manage to put a really stoned guy into a deep trance, after many attempts. Unfortunately the work we tried to do once he was hypnotized was completely ineffective because I was battling mental forces I have not been trained for! Other drugs are mainly stimulants and it's pointless to try.

## Light and Dark

It doesn't really matter how light or dark your environment is, though given the choice I would always prefer to use hypnosis in a darker room. You may have to open and close your eyes a number of times during the process, and if the room is bright this can tend to kick you out of trance more quickly, because of the contrast when you open your eyes to the light. How dark is really a matter of personal preference. During the day you should close your shades or blinds so that there is still natural light in the room, but no bright light source. If you are practicing in the evening, a side-lamp is better than a bright ceiling lamp. Try to make sure it's out of your line of sight.

That's just about it for your environment. Most of these tips are obvious, but they all combine to create the most conducive situation for you to succeed at Self-Hypnosis, so try to consider each one in terms of its practicality for you.

So, you've got your script ready, and you're seated and relaxed in a comfortable, private environment. You're all set, so let's get on with the first exercise.

# Exercise 1 – Simple Induction

The script we are going to use is called 'Master Self-Hypnosis: Simple Induction and Emerge' and in case you have forgotten it can be found using the first link in your e-mail.

## What You'll Be Doing

In this first exercise, we're going to use a standard hypnosis induction to get you used to how hypnosis works.

If you have visited a professional hypnotherapist in the past, it's possible that the 'induction' part of your session may have been quite a prolonged affair. Many therapists use a technique called 'progressive relaxation' to take you gradually into a light trance, and then slowly deepen the state over anything up to an hour. This works fine for most people, but it takes a long time.

## Rapid Induction

A famous American hypnotherapist, Dave Elman, having observed the apparent need to repeat this long-winded conditioning exercise, developed a very successful alternative which accelerates the induction process. I have been using this 'Elman Induction' with hypnosis clients for several years, and found that it works every time. This induction compresses the repetitive conditioning into a series of brief 'mini-inductions' which start to induce a trance, then 'wake up' the subject, before repeating the process again and again. The technique ensures that each time the subject opens his or her eyes, then drops back towards the trance state, they go deeper. The result is a nicely hypnotized subject in a matter of a few short minutes. This is the technique we will be using in our Stage One Exercise.

## Deepening Your Trance

Once this part of the induction is completed, we will use what is known as the 'Escalator' technique to deepen the trance. Again, this is a short procedure, which involves visualising a descent towards what we can call your 'Basement of Relaxation' where both mind and body are fully relaxed. In this first exercise, this 'basement' is where we will rest for a few minutes, and allow you to explore the sensations and clarity which hypnosis offers. At the beginning of this pause you will be offered suggestions of things you can do, however what is most important is that you take time to enjoy the tranquility of the hypnotic state. You will not be expected to make any earth-shattering discoveries at first, however each time you repeat this exercise you will find that you will become more confident and inquisitive.

Whilst you are in this 'Basement of Relaxation' you may find that you can begin to visualise scenes, places, or events. Alternately you may experience feelings, which can often become quite intense. How you experience hypnosis will depend on you as an individual, whether you are principally visual, auditory or kinaesthetic by nature, or maybe a combination of any or all of these.

After an appropriate period of quiet time, the script will begin again and you will be gently emerged from your trance state, until you are wide awake, back in the room, and feeling great.

## During Your Trance

Hypnosis is completely safe and you will never lose your ability to wake yourself up should you feel uncomfortable with what is going on. The likelihood is that you'll wonder about this sometime during your experience, but you will feel so good that you won't feel the need to try to wake yourself up. I invite you to test this for yourself once you have gone through the induction stage.

There are three accepted 'Levels' of hypnotic trance which most professional hypnotherapists use. For the purpose of this explanation, we'll call them Light, Medium, and Deep. In professional practice, the deep state is often used for treating really serious psychological conditions, as well as medical and dental anesthesia.

It is unlikely that you will ever reach a state of Deep ('Comatose') hypnotic trance using Self-Hypnosis. Even if you do, the techniques contained in these scripts will work in exactly the same way, to emerge you back to your full waking state when it's time.

In this Stage One exercise, we'll be targeting the *Light* state. In this state, most people remain fully aware of where they are and what is going on around them, but they choose to 'switch off' that consciousness and 'go inside' to explore their own internal thoughts, images and feelings. You may achieve this Light state on your very first attempt. You may even recognize it when it happens, or you may perhaps feel that nothing has changed, and you're just relaxing in a chair with your eyes closed. It doesn't matter, because you're going to repeat the same exercise several times, and each time you go into hypnosis you will go deeper than the last time, and you'll find new sensations and experiences which will encourage you to go further.

Remember, it's a *conditioning* process, and the more often you do it the better you will become.

When you emerge from your first hypnotic experience, we're going to conduct a little 'de-brief' so that you can reflect on how you got on.

So, make yourself comfortable, put on your headphones, and when you're ready, start the recording.


(Play the Script)


Welcome back! How was that for you? Why don't you have a stretch now, I'm sure you feel like one. You completed the exercise really well. Now just take moment to reflect on what happened.

You might remember everything, or you might remember nothing at all. It may have seemed like a really short time, or alternately you might feel like you've been gone for ages. I can tell you that the whole exercise took less than fifteen minutes.

When you are completely ready, you are going to start the recording again, and repeat the experience, but this time you will easily go much deeper into hypnosis, and each time that you do this you will be able to go deeper still. Right now I suggest you get up and walk around for a few minutes, maybe have a cup of tea or a glass of water. Remember, no coffee and preferably no smoking! Then when you are ready to try it again, come back and make yourself comfortable.

## De-Briefing Yourself

After the first time you try the Exercise, there may be things that you noticed which you can change, in order to make it easier next time. Just run through the checklist below, and make any adjustments before the next repetition.

- Temperature: was I too warm or too cold?
- Comfort: how was my seating position, the position of my hands, and so on?
- Volume: was the recording too loud, too soft?
- Brightness: do I need to lighten or darken the room?
- External sounds: was I distracted? Do I need to stop anything, close any windows, and so on?

These are mainly small things, but any one of them can detract from the overall experience, so it's really worth taking a little time to get everything right, so that there are no obstacles to you achieving that wonderful depth of relaxation which hypnosis offers.

You can go on repeating this Exercise as many times as you like! You will be the best person to judge how well it is working for you, and you will notice the progressive conditioning as you try it again, and again. Although my voice is guiding you, the actual hypnosis is coming from you. You are allowing it to happen, and it is happening. That's the essence of Self-Hypnosis.

You should not think about moving on until you are entirely comfortable with this first exercise. Many people report that the second time they do it, it's much more effective than the first, and this is the conditioning effect we discussed earlier. Just keep repeating the recording as many times as you like. There's no such thing as too much practice!

At some point whilst you are between 'sessions' in this first exercise, it may be useful to ask yourself if this is having any effect on your attitude to stress. It's not so much that you achieve a quick-fix, but instead that you begin to understand how this kind of relaxation technique can be a positive thing for you. You're looking for Potential, and once you appreciate that, you'll find it much easier (and even exciting) to commit to continuing with the process. As I mentioned at the beginning of the book, over 75% of the people who access the first Script go on to complete the whole course.

Next, in Stage Two, we're going to use the skills that you have developed in Stage One to train you how to achieve the hypnotic state on your own.

# Exercise 2 - Sound and Vision

Welcome back. I hope you had a nice break!

Next, we're going to take the skills you developed in Stage One and use them to identify what we call your 'modality', that is to say the PRIMARY way that you experience things in hypnosis. You've already proven that you can easily enter trance, and you've experienced the pleasure of the hypnotic state. Now we will try an exercise to determine if you are primarily Visual (sight), Auditory (sound), or Kinaesthetic (feelings and sensations)

## Script Two: A Day at the Beach

We will use another recorded script which starts off with the same rapid induction we used in Stage One. Once you are in trance, you will be given a Trigger Word, which is 'BEACH' and your task is to experience everything associated with being at a beach. The idea is to 'calibrate' you so that you will be able to tell if you are predominately Visual, Auditory or Kinaesthetic. How you experience the Beach will determine what we call your 'Modality' and this will then be the primary way that you will approach specific exercises whilst in hypnosis.

You will be using your powerful imagination, which is allowing you to roam freely in hypnosis. If you are primarily visual, you may be able to generate a clear image of the beach scene, and to be able to describe it, either during the trance or afterwards. Maybe you will be primarily auditory, in which case you may hear the sounds of the waves, or children playing in the sand. Alternatively, if you are primarily kinaesthetic, you might feel the breeze on your face, or smell the salty air. It's entirely possible that you may experience more than one of these modalities, which is great, however what is important is to find out which is the dominant sense, so that you can then utilize it in future Self-Hypnosis.

I've used the Beach visualisation may times myself. My favourite scenario is to imagine myself at a sophisticated beach bar, sipping an ice cold beer and watching the people sunbathing and swimming. You will develop your own version of 'Beach' and you may find it strangely addictive as an escape from daily life!

The link for the script is the second one in the e-mail.

It's "Exercise Two: Self-Calibration" which you can download or stream just the same as the first one. Much of the script will be familiar to you, which should help you to drop into trance very easily. However, some of the parts are shortened because you simply don't need all the induction techniques, now that you've become proficient. Once you have the Script, make yourself comfortable and quickly run through the checklist below;

- Switch your phone to 'Flight Mode' if you've downloaded the script. If you are going to stream it (over Wi-Fi) select the setting which leaves the Wi-Fi on but turns calls and text messages off.

- Make sure you won't be disturbed for around half an hour.
- Visit the bathroom if you need to.
- Take a few moments to acclimatize yourself to any sounds that you may hear during the Exercise, and explain to yourself that these will not disturb you.

When you are completely ready, start the recording and enjoy the trance!

(Play the Script)

Welcome Back. I hope you had a nice time at the beach! Take a stretch and grab the book, so that we can review what just happened.

## De-Brief

If you followed the preparation instructions and stuck to the recorded script, you should be quite amazed by now at your own ability to enter trance, and what you can do whilst you're there. The Beach Scene usually evokes powerful imagery or sensations in everyone who tries this exercise, and I'm sure you experienced that too. If, for some reason, it wasn't as vivid or literal as you had hoped, don't worry, just repeat the script again, even two or three times, and the effect will increase as you get more proficient at exercising your powerful imagination.

You'll remember from the introduction that this was called a 'Calibration Exercise' and the idea was to try to discover your modality, that is to say are you predominately Visual, Auditory or Kinaesthetic. Your experience at the beach should have given you a good idea of this.

Did you see the colors? Were they bright or dull? Did you see movement or was it like a post-card? If any of these statements are true for you, make a mental note of the answers so that you can build your future visualizations around your strengths.

Maybe you didn't see much, but you heard the sounds. Could you hear the waves, the seagulls, the people talking and kids playing? Maybe you heard a more elaborate sound-track like a beach bar or a restaurant with music. Again, try to recall what you were hearing and make a mental note of how vivid it was, how complex and/or realistic the experience.

Or maybe you mainly felt things, like breeze, smell, or texture? Maybe what you experienced was an 'impression' of the beach, enough to convince you that you were there, even though you couldn't see or hear very much? That's called Kinaesthetic.

You should now be able to assess and decide your dominant Modality. If you can't do it yet, I suggest you run the recording again, now that you know what to expect, and spend some more time at the beach!

You will have accomplished this part of the mission when you are able to say to yourself: "I am Visual/Auditory/Kinaesthetic" Remember, you don't have to have only ONE modality, but you should try to identify your dominant one, because that is the way that you will design your exercises when you start doing more interesting things in your trances.

There is a second use for this beach-scene trance, which you can use for yourself once you've completed all the exercises. You can denominate it your 'Happy Place', and any time you feel stressed, you have a place to go where you can do nothing other than relax. Once you've mastered this technique, you might choose a different scene, such as a Garden, a Mountain Landscape, or anything else that floats your boat. Even a boat!

By now you should be dropping easily into trance, and you should be totally confident in your own ability. You can completely let go and enjoy the experience, and you should also have convinced yourself that each time you do it, you go deeper.

Take a break. In the next chapter, we are going to install the Self-Hypnosis *post-hypnotic suggestion*, so that you will add instant Self-Hypnosis to your rapidly increasing skill-set.

# Exercise 3 - Installing Self Hypnosis

Next, we will use yet another script which is designed to 'install' the process for you to start to self-hypnotize. Again, we'll use a short induction to get you into trance, which you should be finding very easy by now. Once you're in the hypnotic state, you'll be given a series of instructions about how to prepare yourself the next time you want to enter hypnosis, and you'll be invited to experience these simple steps according to the modality we established in the previous exercise. You'll also give yourself a 'post-hypnotic suggestion' which is a memorable Cue Word to use each time you want to go quickly into trance.

## Choosing Your Cue Word

This post-hypnotic suggestion is a powerful device, so you need to choose a cue word or short phrase which is not in regular daily use. The last thing you want is to find yourself drifting into hypnotic trance in the middle of a normal conversation or whilst listening to the radio because someone inadvertently used your cue-word! Using this trigger or word yourself as a cue to enter hypnosis will become a habit, and the more you use it, the easier and more effective it will become. Personally, I use *"And.... Descend!"* as my own cue word, whenever I want to go into trance. You can use this one (unless you're a submariner or a pilot of course) or you can choose one of your own: it really doesn't matter. Just make sure it's unique to you.

Once we've installed the Self-Hypnosis technique in you, and you've implanted your Cue Word, you'll emerge from hypnosis feeling wide-awake as before, and knowing that you now have everything you need to go deeper into hypnosis any time and every time you choose.

Afterwards we can put the training scripts to one side, and you can start practicing Self-Hypnosis for real. Remember, the more often you use it, the better you'll become, so you can simply repeat going in and out of trance as often as you like.

You'll be given some pointers on things that you might like to try whilst you're in self-induced trance, so that you can find out how easy or hard it is to give yourself suggestions. Some people are able to carry quite complex procedures into the hypnotic state. Others use it only for very simple 'one-liners' to address things like focus and concentration, motivation, calmness and so on. And if neither of these things appeals to you, you may be one of those people who simply want to use Self-Hypnosis for recreation or relaxation.

As I said at the beginning of this book, it is perfectly possible to teach yourself some form of Self-Hypnosis just by reading some written instructions. However it's a lot quicker and more effective if you have some help. It's very common for a Professional Hypnotherapist to 'install' Self-Hypnosis when you visit him or her for any reason. We are going to use exactly the same method, but you can expect it to be even more effective because of the time you have already spent becoming confident and familiar with the hypnosis process itself. Let's just run a quick check over what we've done, and what you've achieved so far.

In Stage One, you were induced by script into deepening states of trance. If you followed the system correctly, you will have experienced an increasingly deep and pleasant state of hypnosis, as you repeated the exercise over and over. The key objective of this exercise was to prove to yourself that you are fully capable of entering into and emerging from hypnotic trance, and that the more often you do it, the better and easier it becomes for you.

In the Second Exercise, you once again went into trance using a recorded script, and you imagined being at the beach. This was firstly to demonstrate to you the power of your imagination: that is your ability to create realistic situations and experiences whilst you are in the hypnotic state, and also the practical calibration to find out if you are predominately visual, auditory or kinaesthetic. Knowing this about yourself will help you a lot if and when you start to use your Self-Hypnosis skills for specific purposes later on.

You are now ready to receive the great wisdom that brought you here in the first place!

## How It Will Work

In this exercise, we are going to place you in trance – much more quickly this time – and install the simple skills to enable you to self-hypnotize without the use of recorded scripts. This is really easy, and it won't take long. Once you emerge from this trance, you will have everything you need to start practicing Self-Hypnosis without my help.

First, you need another script, which is the third link in your e-mail. It's called 'Exercise Three: Installing Self-Hypnosis'

Once you have mastered this technique, you will have an 'escape route' which you will be able to use whenever a stressful situation arises. You might think that you need to sit down and close your eyes to become hypnotized, but that is not necessarily the case. With practice, you can use this technique anywhere, anytime, and you won't even need to close your eyes. You will simply use the self-hypnosis technique to cause your body and mind to relax instantly, and choke off the flow of stress-inducing chemicals in your brain and body.

## Remember Your Cue-Word

In a moment you are going to make yourself comfortable, run through the usual check-list, and prepare to be hypnotized again. However, before you start to relax this time, you need to select your Cue-Word which you will be using in the future to start the Self-Hypnosis process. You'll remember that I use *"And... Descend!"* as my Cue Word, and you can use it too if you like. Alternately, please choose something for yourself: make it simple, easily memorable, and personal to you. Choose it now, because you will be taking it into the trance with you, ready to use just before you emerge.

Have you chosen it? Good!

So, once we've completed the induction this time, when you've reached the *basement of your relaxation*, you'll be given a series of instructions which you will use in the future when you want to achieve Self-Hypnosis. This set of instructions will be the way that you induce trance in yourself in a similar environment to the one you are currently using with the scripts. In effect, you will have the skills to replace the scripts (although of course you can use the scripts any time you like if you're feeling lazy!). The way that these instructions will be presented will be a kind of 'trance within a trance' where you will be using your imagination to go through the whole process of Self-Hypnosis. By doing it this way, you should be able to experience the sensations of self-induction with total clarity, which will successfully embed the process in your subconscious mind, enabling you to repeat it later with complete confidence and competence.

You will then emerge yourself from Self-Hypnosis, *but only as far as the script-induced trance that you were in before you learned the Self-Hypnosis instructions*. You'll remain deeply hypnotized whilst we give you the post-hypnotic suggestion, so that you can use your chosen cue-word to drop into Self-Hypnosis any time you like. Once that's done, the recorded script will emerge you to your full waking state once more.

The duration of this exercise is around twenty minutes.

So, make yourself comfortable, check all the environmental factors, and prepare yourself to be hypnotized one more time.

(Play the Script)

And... Stretch!

## De-Brief

So, what we did there was have you go through the procedure of hypnotizing yourself, whilst you were already in hypnosis. If this sounds a little strange to you, don't worry. This method works very well, because it teaches you the simple steps that you'll be using yourself. However by doing it whilst you are already in trance, the instructions are accepted by your subconscious mind without question, so that when you come to execute the procedure for yourself from the normal waking state, you will automatically know that it is going to work and you will have total confidence in your ability to achieve an excellent state of trance all by yourself.

## Practicing Self-Hypnosis

Next, you're going to use what you just learned and practice hypnotizing yourself for the first time.

Here's a reminder of the steps you will take;

Seat yourself comfortably and run through your check-list to make sure you won't be disturbed or distracted.

Listen for any external sounds and accept them, telling yourself that these sounds will not disturb you during your trance.

Think about what you would like to do once you are in trance. Maybe you will be taking some silent time to contemplate nothing in particular, just to see where it leads. Or maybe you have a specific topic you would like to take a look at whilst you're under, in which case try to establish how you will start that process, using either a well-formed image or an internal description of a feeling or sentiment. We'll talk more about this later, but for now, just give yourself a simple starting point that you will be able to use once you're ready. Pictures are good.

Tell yourself that you are ready to enter hypnosis and that when you are finished you will be ready to come out again and feel great. You can speak this aloud or silently say it to yourself.

When you are ready, take a deep breath, hold it for a few moments, and as you exhale, say your Cue Word and close your eyes.

Start to count down from ten, synchronizing the counting with your breathing, so that with every breath you exhale, you double your physical and mental relaxation and go deeper inside.

When you have counted down to one, you will instinctively know if you have fully relaxed your body and mind. If you feel you need to go deeper, use the escalator visualisation that we did in the previous exercises. Go down as many levels as you want, always telling yourself that as you descend, you will be going ever deeper into that wonderful trance state. You will remain completely aware of your own thoughts; however you can detach your mind from your body and leave your physical self on any of the levels until you are ready to come back.

When you have reached the basement of your relaxation, simply rest there for as long as you like. You can drift aimlessly if that is your desire. Or you can bring up the image or trigger for the subject you want to examine, and just allow your mind to explore it. Don't try to force questions and answers, because if you have followed the instructions you will be in a relatively deep state of hypnosis and your imagination will do the work.

When you know that you have gone as far as you need or want in this session, tell yourself that you are ready to emerge from hypnosis and that you can come back any time you want, and go even deeper each time. Start to count upwards, slowly, from one to three. With each number, feel yourself becoming more alert, your physical sensations returning, then your mood clearing, and finally open your eyes feeling refreshed and positive.

Always take a few moments to review what happened, and take a stretch. Don't get up too quickly, because you may have slowed your heart-rate and it might take a few moments for your circulation to come back up to speed.

Once you have this process automated, you can start to speed things up. You'll find that the use of your cue word will take you into a state of deep relaxation quicker each time you use it, and once you know that you can do this anytime, anywhere, you will have a powerful weapon at your disposal which you can activate any time you feel stress or anxiety rising.

Simple, isn't it! Well, it's simple for you, because you took the time and put in the work to go through the conditioning exercises. As I said at the very beginning, the more often you go into hypnosis, the easier and quicker it becomes, and the deeper you are able to descend.

It may look like there's a lot to remember, but there really isn't. All along, I've tried to explain what to expect and what will happen so that you have a good understanding of the hypnotic process, and that's about maintaining your confidence and belief in the efficacy. But if you want a simple step-by-step version of the instructions above, try this;

## Self-Hypnosis Check-List

- Get ready
- Visualize your objective.
- Say that you're ready to go into trance.
- Breathe in, breath out, say your cue word and close your eyes.
- Count down from ten to one and push out the tension so you relax completely.
- Use all your tools to go as deep as you want.
- When you're deep enough, trigger your objective image. Do what you need to do.
- Decide when you're finished, count from one up to three and emerge refreshed.

- Stretch, review, and plan your next adventure!

# Exercise 4 - Ultra Height ®

You have now completed the "Master Self-Hypnosis in a Weekend" training, and you have equipped yourself with a powerful new skill that you can use in many ways. Primarily, you should use the quick Self-Hypnosis technique whenever you feel stress rising, so you can get a holistic time-out to calm yourself, shut off the chemicals, and put yourself in a better position to deal with the challenge.

For many people, that's enough. You may feel that you have what you need for tactical intervention.

However, for others, there is a need to delve deeper into self-examination, to look for new ideas and solutions to old problems and issues. Allow me to introduce you to the wonder that is Ultra Height ®.

Ultra Height is an hypnotic technique pioneered, trained and licensed by Gerry Kine, the renowned US hypnotherapist, at the Omni Hypnosis center in Florida. It involves the induction of a deeper trance state, with a new twist. The objective of Ultra Height is to place you in a "white space of purity", shutting off all external sensations so that you use your mind 100%.

To understand Ultra-Height, and the joyful state it induces, you really need to try it for yourself. It requires a well-practiced visualisation ability, so it should only be attempted once you are completely happy with the previous three exercises.

The induction is designed to enable you to 'uncouple' your body and your mind, then allow your mind to rise high into (some describe it as) 'cloud-space' where you can wander round and examine yourself from the inside. People report discovering answers to long-standing questions, directions about where to head next, and other things like this. I have used it myself many times and it has always been a thoroughly refreshing and energizing experience.

In the context of stress, this is the pointy end of 'Massive Action' which will be explained in the final section of the book. The idea is that you can go to a place where the petty distractions of everyday life are temporarily removed from your decision process, so that you can focus only on your own happiness and well-being. If you can achieve this, it could enable you to see more clearly the direction you would like your life to take, without the earth-bound obstacles that may be obscuring your view.

Of course, like all modern hypnosis, Ultra Height is completely safe. However, it can be a powerful experience, so be prepared to arrive back with some different ways of thinking about things. You need to know that before you commit to it. Once more, the more you try it, the more successful you will become.

So, set aside an hour, and run through your checklist, and when you're ready to begin, the Script is the fourth link in your e-mail, called (unsurprisingly) "Ultra Height". There's a short introduction before the trance begins, and there's a de-brief afterwards.

Enjoy....

(Play the Script)

# Section 4 – Massive Action

So, to recap; in the first section you learned about the physiological effects of stress, and why it presents such a clear and present danger to your long-term health and well-being. Hopefully you took the opportunity to evaluate the role of stress in your own life (or maybe the role of your life in your own stress!) and concluded, as any sane person would, that you really must get to grips with stress before it starts to seriously hurt you and those around you.

Next, in section 2, we examined the more conventional approaches to stress reduction and stress management. All of these have a valid place in your armory, and some will work better than others for each individual case. It's entirely possible that you found something in there which works well for you, and because stress is essentially mentally generated, there's an argument that 'belief in a ritual' may indeed provide the relief you seek. If that is the case, I wish you well and encourage you to experiment with the various methods to see what combination helps you best.

In section 3, you experienced Hypnosis. If you did this correctly (please don't skim over the exercises, because repetitive conditioning significantly amplifies the effect) you will have begun to experience some levels of peace and tranquillity, which is at the opposite end of the scale to the stress condition, and hence may turn out to be your personal panacea. If you completed Exercise 3, you already have an excellent way to activate the relaxation response, which will in turn switch off your stress-chemical generators. Your new ability to drop yourself quickly into trance (which can certainly include keeping your eyes open) will really help you to cope much better with 'tactical' stress situations as and when they arise. You can take this self-hypnosis to untold heights of success if you practice often, and experiment with different situations.

At the end of Section 3, you tried Ultra-Height hypnosis. Only you can know how this worked out for you. When I have used it with real-live clients, every single one has reported something out of the ordinary. In each case, the effect has been overwhelmingly positive. I did once have a client who actually experienced motion sickness during the final descent phase. Although it was unpleasant for her at the time, she came back for another go, because she understood the negative effect was actually a validation of how well it had worked for her. That the manifestation of physical symptoms derived from an entirely mental process was validation of the power of the technique, in her case.

All of these techniques and interventions so far may be summarized as 'stress reduction' or 'stress management' tools. If you have found a combination which satisfies your requirements, then congratulations, and I hope you go on to live a happier and less stressful life in the future.

However for some people, that simply isn't enough! Merely coping or suppressing the stress may not satisfy your objectives. None of the techniques are locked in or permanent and you should plan to practice, review, and refresh your toolkit at regular intervals if you want to prevent yourself from regressing to the earlier state.

So, now we come to "Massive Action".

Massive Action is an approach to what we will call 'Situational Stress'. Many people find themselves locked into a personal situation which is unsatisfactory, and which generates stress in and of itself. Situations such as career, relationships, health concerns and finances can bring about what seems to be an insoluble set of circumstances. You may be trapped, even if you don't immediately recognize it as such, and from the inside of your dungeon you may not be able to see a practical way out. It's important to know that there is always a solution to every problem, but you may require a shift in mind-set to be able to escape.

No-one is born to be unhappy, but where and when you find yourself may be initially outside your control. The principle behind Massive Action is to recognize your situation, then change it.

Many people are terrified by the concept of change, because it takes them into new and unfamiliar territory, with all the incumbent questions about whether they will (a) be able to achieve a change, and (b) what will happen to them once they reach their new situation.

The axiom is that the situation you are in is causing stress, which will ultimately self-perpetuate and make your life worse. Who would want that?

Finally, before we examine the main Chronic Stress situations, be prepared. At the beginning of this book, I explained that we would take a 'brutal' approach to stress-elimination. You may have been wondering when that would happen, because the previous three sections have been relatively gentle on you. Please remember that this book is for men, but the scenarios could equally apply to women if the roles were to be reversed.

Here begins the brutality!

## Situational Stress

So far, we've been concentrating on tactics and strategies to help you deal with the symptoms of stress. It may be that your own stress is caused by circumstances which you cannot control, or that you *think* you cannot control.

In this section we will look at the two main underlying causes of controllable stress; your Work, and your Relationship. Of course, you might say that your stress is financial, but I would argue that finances are almost invariably a product of one of these two main situations.

Massive Action is about changing things, not just at a detail level, but wholesale re-organisation of the way you live your life. If you change the situation which creates the stress, you have a very good chance of removing the stress completely. At source.

# Work Induced Stress

'Working on the Chain Gang, Going Down, Down, Down!'

### "I Hate My Job"

So, who doesn't? Frankly, having to work at all is not much fun for most people. Trouble is, if you don't go to work, you'd never leave the house, so you're probably stuck with it, at least for a while. Workplace stress is a catastrophic social anomaly, costing billions each year in just about every country. Deaths, riots, and revolutions are often the end product of unresolved workplace stress issue. On an individual level, it can totally cripple some people. If you're heading in that direction, you need to head it off, and quickly.

## Work Related Stress

Work-related stress is probably the most common type of stress. In many cases, the problems arise from interpersonal relationships, and are often born of poor communication. Other people are simply in the wrong job, for which there can be many reasons.

According to the American Institute of Stress, numerous studies show that work stress is far and away the major source of stress for American adults, and it is climbing progressively. The common factor seems to be a perception of having diminished control but increased demands. These factors have been demonstrated to contribute to increased rates of heart attack, hypertension (high blood pressure) and many other disorders. Remarkably, in some major US cities, the relationship between work stress and heart attacks is so well acknowledged that police officers who suffer coronary events such as heart attacks, either whilst working or off duty, are automatically assumed to have suffered a work-related injury. Compensation schemes are in place, which include heart-attacks suffered whilst fishing on vacation, or gambling in Las Vegas!

Of course different occupations bring different kinds of stress. For someone who thrives on demanding challenges, the prospect of working on a dull assembly-line kind of job could be the thing that would stress them the most. Alternately, some people of a gentler disposition would be unsuited to a front-line public-facing challenge such as the police, or a high school teacher working in the inner city.

The obscuring fact is that there are thousands of people who are able to work without stress problems in these occupations, which just underlines the fact that we are all different, and it is our own uniqueness which determines how we will deal with particular situations. Stress is a highly personalized phenomenon and can vary widely, even in identical situations for different reasons. One survey showed that having to complete paperwork was more stressful to many police officers than the dangers associated with pursuing criminals!

In notable studies conducted in the USA, the extent of stress in the workplace is quite startling (sources: The National Institute for Occupational Safety and Health, Harris Interactive; Attitudes in the American Workplace Seven)

- 40% of workers reported their job was very or extremely stressful.
- 25% view their jobs as the number one stressor in their lives.
- 26% of workers said they were often or very often burned out or stressed by their work. An amazing 80% of workers feel stress on the job, and nearly half say they need help in learning how to manage stress.
- 42% of workers said their co-workers needed such help.
- 25% felt like screaming or shouting because of job stress.

Workplace stress even coined a phrase "Going Postal" following a series of incidents between 1986 and 1997 when more than 40 people were shot dead in incidences of workplace rage in the United States Postal Service.

The common thread running through these case studies are twofold: in the first place the primary stress or for each of the subjects appears to be the way that they were being managed. This could be either an individual or a company problem. Of course, there are procedures and protocols to deal with incompetence and bullying in the workplace, although people are often not inclined to seek redress via these routes unless they have the backing of a union body. Not everyone is so fortunate.

But the real underlying issue is that, irrespective of whether a company takes action against an individual manager or fixes a system which is causing stress amongst its workers, people are simply afraid of losing their jobs. When caught up in a stress situation at work, the immediate solution which springs to mind is always to change one's situation, however when you're right up against the coal face, the only change that appears to be viable is a change of job, and that is often much more complex than it sounds.

So, what else can you do about it? For men, there is the added difficulty of inherent machismo preventing them from confessing any problems. We are hardwired to avoid any display of perceived weakness, for fear that it will damage our position in the herd. Although there are formal ways to deal with stress in industrial situation, it's not always easy to take that first step.

With this in mind, it may be very useful to develop strategies of your own, in private, which enable you to reduce the negative effects that these external factors are having on your life, your performance, and your happiness. You can now call on your Self-Hypnosis skills to relax yourself whenever stress arises.

Use my 'Brutal Truth' method. When you encounter a stressful situation, before you allow yourself to be drawn into that dangerous stress cycle, remind yourself that an external situation is threatening your health if you permit it, and simply use every tool at your disposal not to allow it.

# Massive Action in the Workplace

The problem for most people is that they're locked into a financial model which gives them no room to breathe. Wage slavery is a bitch, and sooner or later you have to get on top of it, or you've got decades of pain ahead of you. If you're the family breadwinner, you are carrying the added stress of having to provide a home and security for your family. That's the way boys are brought up, and before you know it you're forty or fifty years old and you just haven't done anything for yourself!

The trouble for many men is that in the absence of any other highlights in our lives, we allow our work to define us. Common sense tells us that's the wrong way to live, but nevertheless it happens.

Men are brought up in the West to believe that job and career are the most important facets of their existence. In truth, this is just a modification of the purpose of life itself. If you don't have a job, if you don't earn a living, and you are not respected by at least a small group of people, you can't attract women and therefore you're not going get any sex. No Money, No Honey! Sooner or later, the human race will die out completely and the whole shebang will have been a monumental waste of a few million years!

We'll be looking more detail at the stresses that come from relationships later, but unless you are bringing home the bacon, it's going to be a tricky feat to sustain any kind of intimate relationship, and that is a key element in your hierarchy of needs!

So what often tends to happen is that we lock ourselves into unfulfilling careers and unsatisfactory occupations simply in order to maintain the stability of our lives in general. There's a huge stigma attached to idleness and unemployment, and with few exceptions nobody wants to find himself in this situation. Welfare sucks!

When you think about the sources of workplace stress, it may be all too easy to say "if only I earned twice as much money, I would be happy". It's hard to deny that more money generally improves things, but it's also the case that extremely highly paid people often suffer professional stress the worst.

So the first question you have to ask yourself is, from a financial standpoint, do you have enough? Is your life and indeed your survival being compromised by poor pay? If the answer to the second question is yes, then clearly your situation is unsustainable. If you are locked into a rigid workplace system which does not reward you on the basis of merit, then now is the time to realize that you have little option but to change your situation.

Here I like to use a motto called 'Just Do SOMETHING!" It's a really simple formula that states that your stress reduces significantly the moment you decide to do something about your situation.

In physiological terms, anxiety and excitement are closely related. It is the context (whether it is predominately negative or positive) which determines how we experience the chemical reactions. So if you replace the frustration of a locked-in situation with the anticipation of an undefined but different future, you can change the negative of anxiety (stress) into a positive (excitement).

The simplest solution to an unsatisfactory work or career situation is to change it. You are allowed to do that, you know! If anyone tells you different, they are either lying, coercing, or bullying you.

Are you having problems with your workmates, your boss, or anyone else associated with your job? Taking an objective view for a moment, even in your wildest dreams can you see a way to improve your work relationships? If you can, then you need to make a plan and execute it. If you can't, then again you need to take massive action and change your situation.

So, when it comes to fixing workplace stress, you have a limited range of options available to you:

- Implement personal strategies which will negate any or all of the pressures which are causing your workplace stress;
- Adopt a portfolio of stress management techniques. This assumes that you cannot change the situation, but you may be able to adapt and modify your response to the stressors;
- Plan and execute an escape strategy to get yourself out of the situation and leave the stress behind you.

The first option requires two things on your part: firstly, you need to audit your situation objectively, and identify the specific factors which are acting as stressors in your workplace environment. You may not feel able to do this on your own, in which case you should co-opt a trusted friend or colleague to assist you. Remember, there's no use complaining if no one's listening, and in any case it won't get any better unless you take some positive action.

The objective with this process, once you've identified the key issues, starts with a simple decision. Now you have all these factors written down in front of you, do you believe that you have a fighting chance of fixing at least half of them? If not, you need to adopt the second or third options. If you see a list of things which can reasonably be changed or adapted, then the next step is to divide them into internal and external lists. The internal list is the list of things you can do, using the weapons that are at your disposal, to modify your approach to each factor and gain control over it so that it no longer exerts a stress trigger on you.

## Dealing with Procrastination

For example (and this is one of the biggest factors in any workplace stress) are you exercising procrastination? Is the combination of factors causing you to self-defeat, which inevitably causes your workload to build up towards the end of the day, the end of the week, or the end of the month? A typical symptom of chronic workplace stress is introspection and over-analysis during the working day. You look at the pile of paper in front of you, and even though you may be perfectly capable of clearing it within the time allotted, you put off starting it because you know you simply don't enjoy the task. The end result is that the pile that was there on

Monday is still there on Thursday, and maybe even grew a little. So now you have two days to do the work that you should have done in five. So you worry for three days, and then you're overloaded for two! When you think about it like that it doesn't make much sense, does it? And this is something you can easily change in yourself, provided that you view the change as part of an overall plan to improve your situation.

Procrastination is one of those things that you should be able to handle with your new Self-Hypnosis skills. Try setting aside half an hour each evening for just one week, and putting yourself into trance. Use a one-liner such as: "The earlier I start, the earlier I'll finish."

I'm not a great believer in a "workbook" approach to self-help because nobody really wants to do the exercises, so you lose interest in the book before it even gets to the meaty part. So I'm not going to suggest a list of things that you should identify, but instead encourage you to brainstorm freely and produce one of your own. Everyone is different, every work environment has its own uniqueness and idiosyncrasies, and you are best placed to know what is pissing you off.

However I would like to pay some attention to one very common factor suffered by stressed workers and executives.

## Too Many Hours at Work

Do you find yourself going to work earlier and earlier, and potentially staying later and later in the evening? If you are falling into this trap, you need to identify why you are doing it. You may have convinced yourself that it's the only way you can cope with your workload, but I'm guessing that's probably not the real reason. Going in early may be simply because you need quiet time before everyone else arrives at the office or the factory. But seriously, are you actually achieving anything extra by doing this? There is an argument that says that you might be beating the traffic or avoiding the rush on public transport, in which case this might be an entirely healthy habit. But alternately are you simply going in early so that others in your workplace have an impression that you are more committed, or work harder than they do? This is a symptom of workplace competition, which is a huge stressor for some people.

Staying late at the office can have hugely detrimental effects on your personal life, your sleep cycle, and your general well-being. There are 24 hours in every single day, and these logically break down into eight hours sleeping, eight hours for working, and eight hours for doing other things. Modern workplace practices may have caused the eight working hours to extend to nine or ten, and there's nothing intrinsically wrong with this provided you're still getting a reasonable amount of sleep, and enough time to fulfil your personal responsibilities and grab some relaxation time. But if you're showing up to work two hours early, and leaving two or three hours late, that's not good. Nobody ever went to their grave wishing they'd spent more time at the office!

There's a certain kind of manager or director who exerts a subtle expectation that you will stay in the office as late as they do. All that is happening is that they are transferring their own stress situation to you. Maybe their home life is shitty, maybe they don't have any friends, or maybe they can't cope with their own workload! Do you feel unable to pack up your bags and go home at a reasonable time because your boss is still there?

One way out of this spiral of destruction may be to have an honest conversation, and say to him or her that your work/life balance (i.e. your home and family) is critically important to you and has a direct bearing on your effectiveness in the workplace. Perhaps volunteer that you would be willing to work later on one or two evenings a week if that is required of you, and ask which days would be most suitable. By adopting this approach, you are highlighting the issue, which with modern employment law will be very difficult for your manager to side-step, but you're also showing a willingness to be adaptable and versatile in your approach, which unless you're working for a tyrant, will generally come across as a positive and professional approach to something that they may not even have considered. Think about it, does your boss really expect you to be there as late as he is every night, or are you just drawing the inference?

Of course you or he may be avoiding going home because maybe it's even more unpleasant when you get there! In the next chapter we deal with relationships stress.

## Drawing a Line

A really simple way to mark the transition from work to personal time is to adopt a "clear-desk" policy for yourself. Good organisation in every aspect of your life will have a dramatic and positive effect on your stress levels, and nowhere is this truer than in how you handle the end of your work day. If you leave your office with your desk clear and tidy, that not only allows you to make a clear cut-off between the hours spent there and the hours you are not spending there, but also will have a significant calming influence when you walk through the office door the following morning.

And having a clear desk just doesn't involve sweeping everything into a draw and hiding it! You must implement a system where the last half-hour of each working day is spent disposing of spurious paperwork and outstanding small tasks which are within your capabilities to finish before you go home.

This is a physical manifestation of a psychological strategy. If you know that you have finished most if not all of your tasks of the day before you put your coat on, you will not only have cleared your desk, but will have cleared your mind as well. If you leave tasks unfinished because you were poorly organized, then you will take the elements of stress associated with those tasks home with you. Thinking about work when you're not at work is difficult to avoid, but if you want to beat your workplace stress then you should be aiming to have put the day's tasks behind you, so that if you are going to think about work in the evening or the weekend, you are thinking positively about planning and future tasks. This strategy will simply lift you from fear and loathing into a much brighter and more positive frame of mind.

## Workplace Relationships

The issue of workplace relationships looms large in any stress situation. Although there are many different variants there are a few significant categories which are easy to identify.

Do you suffer from, or are you observing bullying in the workplace? The human race has significantly evolved over the last century or so, and bullying is less of a problem now because of the raft of legislation in place to deal with it. Nevertheless, there are still some knuckle-draggers out there who have not adapted to the 21st-century, and will use oppressive tactics, often to deal with their own professional inadequacies. If you are on the receiving end of workplace bullying, you need to suspend any fear that you may have, and address it through the correct channels. If you work for a large organisation, your Human Resources Department will have filing cabinets full of manuals and training courses. No chief executive worth his salt will tolerate bullying in his business, because of the detrimental effects it can have on both internal morale and external image.

In a smaller company it may be less organized, in which case you need to take a discreet and professional approach and go to the top if possible. Most senior managers are fully aware that if an employee decides to take formal action because of a legitimate grievance over workplace conditions, it can tie the company up in expensive and time-consuming processes and litigation, and any boss will be keen to avoid going down such a road.

Therefore if you're going to take this approach, it must be without emotion. You need to approach it via either a formal or informal complaints procedure and have a very clear idea of what it is you want to say, and how you would like it to be dealt with. Explicit threats and coercion will simply alienate the people you need to help you. However if you approach the situation mindfully, that is to say that you are sure of your facts and your rights before you kick off any complaint procedure, you will engender respect and you'll be taken more seriously and treated fairly in most cases. The last thing you want to do is stumble tearfully into the boss's office telling you can't cope because somebody's using your coffee mug! The approach you should take needs to include benefit statements for the company itself, such as "if we can improve the collaboration between Person X and person Y (when one of them may be you) then the efficiency of the Department/Company will improve," the implication being that any improvement in this department will flow to the bottom line.

Perhaps you're suffering from workload issues. Are you in a processing job, i.e. stressed because your department is understaffed and you're being forced to take on more work than you can reasonably achieve? This is a common problem in administrative businesses and is likely responsible for the high turnover of admin staff. Unfortunately, after the financial crisis of the last five or six years, there are more low-skilled people chasing every job and there's no real need or incentive for companies to pay over the odds. Middle management in these types of businesses often tends to be limited, perhaps having risen up from the ranks of the worker bees without any formal management training.

Managers who have not been correctly trained tend to model themselves on what they have observed in the people above them during their careers. If they have seen that people got ahead by being tough and driving for targets, without taking too much notice of the human factors involved, they will inevitably model themselves the same way. Therefore, if you're going to approach such a blunt instrument with such a basic issue, you will need to think carefully about how to dress it up, and how to keep control of yourself whilst you attempt to change the situation. Once again I must stress that taking emotion into an industrial or commercial complaints procedure is wholly counter-productive and rarely achieves a positive result. To you it may be a simple case of "we're understaffed so the work isn't getting done properly" which may be easy for a middle manager to dismiss. However, once again you need to construct your arguments around a set of benefits which they will derive from attending to your complaint. If you can come up with specific instances where inaccuracies in your process business have caused problems, then your manager or superior can be led to understand that their performance and the judgment of it by their higher-ups will be greatly enhanced by them taking on the problem and solving it (on your behalf).

Are your working conditions unacceptable? We've all seen the sweatshops in Bangladesh and Thailand where people sit on cardboard boxes and use machinery with no safety guards! These are extreme examples in the West these days, again because legislation and regulation have evolved to eliminate them. It's a tricky situation if you find yourself in a workplace where your employer is flagrantly ignoring the rules, and unless you are a member of a strong workers union you're unlikely to get much joy in this department. Even self-hypnosis isn't going to help you solve it, so this may be a situation where only Massive Action (change of situation) is going to fix it for you! If your workplace is unsafe or unsavory and this is causing you stress, and you don't have a realistic expectation of getting your employers to modify the situation, you need to get the hell out of there as fast as possible!

## Making the Change

Once you have reconciled your situation, that is to say that you have considered every option available to you in your workplace, and determined that the optimum solution is to leave, then you have choices.

If you're situation is such that only a similar job in a similar organisation is going to work, you need to construct an organized Action Plan to change your employer. Clearly, getting a new job is many times easier if you already have a job, and if you can count on reasonable references from your existing employer, then you should not rock the boat as you move yourself towards that situation.

Take your time. Organize your job search like a military campaign. Set up a system for yourself so that you do something each day to move yourself towards the ultimate goal of finding a more fulfilling occupation. As you already learned earlier in this section, once you make a firm decision to change things, you will immediately start to experience less stress and more hope for the future.

## Get a Great Resume

Get your résumé in shape, but do it privately. If you have never written a résumé before, get some help, particularly on the formatting. Invest in a service; there are hundreds of these online, costing anything from $100 to $1000, and even more if you are a senior executive or a specialist. Some well-regarded services are listed here:

Blue Sky Resumes:
**http://www.blueskyresumes.com/**

Great Resumes Fast:
**http://www.greatresumesfast.com/**

The Resume Centre:
**http://www.theresumecenter.com/**

These organisations produce hundreds of resumes every month, so they know exactly what to put in, and what to leave out. Once you have a professional-looking resume in your hands, you'll feel more confident about approaching agencies and employers. In the current jobs market, getting to interview is the primary objective, and to do this you must have the right tools for the job.

## Hunting Down the Opportunities

Rather than just blasting out applications to every employer in your industry or area, make a shortlist of companies you'd like to work for. Ask your friends and contacts (but not your workmates, obviously) for information and recommendations.

Get yourself a Professional Account on LinkedIn (www.linkedin.com). Over the past few years, LinkedIn has become the platform of choice for many employers seeking new people, because they can use targeted recruitment from as little as $99 a job, massively undercutting the conventional recruitment consultancies. Plus, these jobs are rarely advertised elsewhere. Using the online tools, you can search for jobs and apply directly. There are tens of thousands of jobs on LinkedIn.

Try to think outside the box. It's pointless to move from one company to another if you're going to run into exactly the same situation as you're already in. List your skills, and think about how they may apply to a different industry, and why you might be attractive because of some unique experience or skill-set that you bring.

## Do Your Research

Decide who you want to work for, and research the Company and its Products. When you make your approach, either through LinkedIn, or another online platform, or direct to the corporation itself, you need to have an eye-catching one-liner which tells the reader that you know something useful and can match your skills to their requirement. That's how you'll stand out from the crowd.

## Even More Massive Action

If you go this route, that is to uplift yourself from your stressful professional situation, don't limit yourself. Maybe its time to head out west and learn how to rope cattle. Perhaps serving burgers to the troops in Kabul is going to be more fulfilling than flipping them in a truck-stop in Cincinnati? Sure, you may feel like your existing structure of domestic responsibilities is a restrictive handbrake on your possibilities, but if you allow your limitations to define your future, think about where you're going to be in twenty or thirty years, assuming you're still above ground of course!

The world of work is changing rapidly. Smart people are doing things differently, and thousands of people just like you are taking Massive Action every day to change their situation and reduce their stress. If you have an appetite for new ideas, or maybe you just developed one after reading this section, I recommend two books for you to read.

## 'The Four-Hour Work Week' by Tim Ferris

This is the classic guide on 'Lifestyle Design' and how to free yourself from the corporate structure by doing things differently. And it doesn't only apply to the self-employed (as you might expect) but gives numerous examples about (for example) how to persuade your employer to support remote working, so you end up with more time for yourself. I have personally read this book three times now, and have implemented many of its recommendations. It's a life-changing book which everyone should read before they make decisions about their professional future.

## 'Rework' by Jason Fried & David Heinemeier Hanson

This is a genius manifesto which turns the world of (small to medium-sized) business on its head. In this book you will learn why 80% of what businesses do is next-to-pointless, and will give you oodles of ideas on how to approach things differently. We talked earlier about how to sell benefits of change to your employer, and its equally true that if you are in your own business or at management level in someone else's, there are lots of simple modifications you can make that will lower not only your own stress level, but that of those around you.

# Chapter Summary

Don't accept the status quo. Your work should not define you, at least not exclusively. You are an individual, with your own needs, hot buttons, and dreams/ambitions. You have the right to pursue your life on your own terms. If you are being prevented from doing so, you need to make a change.

Only consider remaining in an unsatisfactory or frustrating professional situation if you are able to form a clear view of how you can change the internal circumstances to reverse and eliminate the stressors.

Clear your desk. Don't work at home, especially not at the weekend.

In any case of industrial dispute, even if you're just dealing with trivia, there is no place for anger or emotion. When you are negotiating from a position of weakness (which is the probable case) you have to be calm and know your onions.

Always seek to reduce your working hours. Nobody ever went to their grave wishing they'd spent more time at the office.

Be prepared to take a backward step if it has a beneficial effect on your stress. Money is very important, but you can't spend anything if you're sick, or worse, dead!

Don't limit yourself. The notion of a single career for life is outdated, and becoming less relevant to modern life. Can you really see yourself doing this for the rest of your working life? Of course not!

Scour the world for new ideas about how you can change your life to fit your desires, rather than just sucking up everything that's dealt to you. There is no rule that says you should be unhappy, so don't be.

# Relationship Stress

## 'Caught in a Bad Romance'

I'm going to unreservedly apologise in advance for the brutal approach I take to this subject. Many, many people sacrifice their life and happiness because of their main relationship. This can be the worst kind of 'locked-in' situation, forcing you to sacrifice any hope of future happiness, and engendering chronic and ever-present stress which will inevitably shorten your useful life. This is what humans do to each other, but you don't have to lie down and take it!

It's impossible to make the rest of your life go well if your home life stinks. Many men screw up early in the piece, by marrying the first woman who gives them regular sex! Trouble at home impacts on every other aspect of your life. You end up taking the stress to work, or into your friendships. You might think that if you stay faithful, stick around, and do the right thing, eventually things will get better. Generally, they don't. A bad relationship usually only gets worse, and no amount of counselling can move you back from a negative position to a positive one. So the stress you feel now can only continue (at best) and increase (at worst).

The main stress inducing factors in a conventional 'partner' relationship are usually:

## Money

Maybe you are over-extended, pe~~r~~
with your mortgage or rent. If you
information with your partner it's prob~~a~~
arguments, and one or other of you may be ~~_
the blame, or at least having to put up with acc~~
of inadequacy or profligacy. So, not only are
permanently stressed by your financial situation, b~~
this is amplified by the additional pressure coming from
your partner, or between you. This type of problem won't
fix itself. Inevitably, this has to change.

## Sex

After money problems, sex is the number two cause of
stress in a relationship. People often use sex as a
currency or "weapon of influence" in their relationships,
and the irony is that men in particular fall for it most of
the time. Alternately, your partner may no longer enjoy
sex, either in general or specifically with you. The self-
help bookshops are packed full of advice, which is always
worthy of consideration, and there are thousands of
therapists out there just waiting to fix you. But after
you've tried all that, and it hasn't worked for you, you
might be forced to face the reality that the excitement of
a healthy and stimulating sexual relationship with your
partner may have run its course. So unless you're
prepared to be unfaithful (not recommended) or celibate
(that's up to you) this might also need to change.

d to the sex issue, it could be that one or other of you longer find the other one attractive. This manifests elf in a loss of respect, or even contempt at the outer mits. It's hard to see a future once a relationship reaches this point, so if she doesn't fancy you any more, that's probably not going to improve. So the situation must change.

Sorry to be brutal, but the recurring theme is "You should love me for me!" But if Me has put on the fat-suit or simply stopped trying to look nice for you, you are trapped! You can't beat human nature. If you've stopped loving your partner because they're just not the person you want to be with any more, ask yourself this; are you willing to spend the remainder of your sorry, compromised life waking up next to someone who you'd rather wasn't there? Is it reasonable that you should compromise your inner-self because your significant other doesn't respect you enough to make an effort to be attractive?

But please, please make sure that you are absolutely blameless before you go down this road. Are you the best you can be?

## Family

A partnership, particularly a marriage, isn't just about the two people concerned. There are family tentacles reaching out (and in) from all directions. Your partner's family may be a problem in your relationship, and simply trying to discuss this, let alone deal with them, may be a huge source of background (chronic) stress. In your head, you may want to say "it's them or me", but the reality is that you know what will happen if you force the issue; you'll come second in the choice. Now, this may be a useful tactic to employ when you want to force the end-game, because it will give you emotional vindication, but equally be aware that you will be pilloried and vilified forever once you're gone, and that may have a disproportionate effect on the relationships your kids enjoy, if you have any. So be careful. Nevertheless, if you can't see your relationship working out because of either family, and you can't change them, you'll probably have to change it.

## Face Facts

Do not be afraid to face the truth. You need to switch on your selfish gene, which is always there but usually suppressed. You are one of a kind, and although society may have conditioned you to believe that you are responsible for everyone else in your immediate circle, that doesn't mean that you should sacrifice your own life and happiness. You are not a beast of burden, and if your relationship is the source of your stress, and is making you feel that way, you have to find a way to change it, which usually means going solo.

Escaping from an inappropriate relationship requires a lot of planning. The last thing you should be doing is sharing your issues with the person who is causing your problems. In fact, discussing it with anyone, including your closest friends, will always bring subjective advice, based on their view of the situation, and it won't help. You need to make your plan (call it a 'fantasy' or 'contingency' if that helps you) and store it away whilst you work out the logistics.

The amazing thing about approaching it in this way is that the minute you change it from just a wish to a potential escape plan, you'll find a lot of your stress will lift.

You'll probably feel that you have to 'do the right thing' and you do. You have to treat your partner with respect and dignity throughout. You're not going to war, because that will just create more stress, which will spread, especially if there are kids involved. You have to map out your course in private, so that when you eventually press the button, assuming that you do, you've ticked all the boxes. Don't share, and definitely don't threaten.

First, identify the issues for yourself, calmly and logically, and name them. Write them down if it helps you to focus, just make sure your list is well hidden. Don't put it on a computer that could be 'hacked', because a vicious or scorned spouse will go to any length to gain an advantage, especially if the situation involves divorce or any other kind of legal machinations. When it comes to lawyers, they're only there to take your money. They won't understand or care about your situation, so they are not the people you want to be confiding in.

Your objective is to remove yourself from the stressful situation with the minimum of collateral damage, and move on with your life, hopefully in a happier place.

## Financial

Many people are constrained from taking the appropriate steps to escape from an inappropriate relationship because of perceived financial factors. Whilst money is important, and is indeed usually at the center of any major decision, it is not as important as happiness. Of course the two can co-exist, and happiness can be elusive if you're really struggling to make ends meet, but everything is relative.

Work out what you can afford to live on, and make that your baseline. It's all you need, because once you're free of the situation, the handbrake will be released and you will soar to greater heights. Everything else you can leave behind.

## Children.

Many people stay locked in a loveless or inappropriate relationship "for the sake of the kids." I'll let you into a secret. Unhappy kids in one unhappy household will ALWAYS do better in two happy households, after an appropriate period of adjustment. You won't damage them, and if you handle the situation correctly, they'll always come back to you. Of course, if your wife or partner decides to be vindictive you'll probably go through a rough time. But if you're smart and well-organized, it needn't be a long-term issue. Kids are smart, and they don't hold grudges for long.

Take a step back and look at your performance as a father (or mother, because although I'm writing this book from a man's perspective, the advice is equally useful for women). With all the stress in your life, and all the stuff that's going on at home, are you really doing the best job for them? Might it not be better for them if you were happy and stress free? Maybe you'll only see them at weekends, but if that's in an environment of fun and love, isn't that better than five nights and the whole weekend of Daddy being overwhelmed and unresponsive? Remember, in a few short years they'll be adults themselves, and the relationship you build with your children once they are old enough to be treated like grown-ups is by far the most rewarding.

## Guilt

Probably the most useless and wasteful of all human emotion is Guilt. What's worse is that Guilt creates additional stress. When relationships go bad, people feel guilty if they start to think that they might be better off on their own, and this especially true if there are children in the mix.

Know this: no situation ever improved by someone feeling guilty. Guilt sucks energy. Time spent pondering the rights and wrongs of your intended actions is simply pointless. Sure, you need to have perspective on the moral position, but you need to shelve guilt and focus on practical remedies.

Another problem with guilt is that it often leads to confession, and that can be seriously dangerous for your health and well-being. If you are in a bad relationship, and you think that confessing your feelings to the other person is going to somehow improve things, you are sadly mistaken, as you will soon find out if you try it. Confession often appears to be a path to absolution, but in this situation it is simply a road to nowhere nice. Everything you do, every action you take, and every plot you hatch must be primarily about moving your life to a better place. You may have moral and/or legal obligations to your partner, your family and so on, but that's where it ends. This is your life we're talking about, and every unnecessary concession you make will be something less that you take with you, so don't.

## How to Leave

This section focused on helping you to face up to reality, and exploring the possibilities of how life might be if you are strong enough to strike out on your own. This is probably the biggest decision you're ever going to make, and I am not particularly qualified to advise you on how to enact it, so I will recommend two more great books that you should absolutely read if you are considering such a course of action:

## 'How to Dump your Wife' by Lee Covington

The main reason I recommend this book is because Lee Covington is a woman! But this lady knows exactly how to talk to men, and her book is a comprehensive deconstruction of the things that can and will happen to you once you start the process of leaving a bad relationship. This book majors on Preparation and

Planning, so that when you eventually throw the switch (assuming you do) you will be meticulously prepared for all the potentially nasty and uncomfortable steps that follow.

## 'The 10 Stupidest Mistakes Men Make When Facing Divorce (and How to Avoid Them)" by Joseph Cordell

Cordell is a highly respected divorce attorney in the USA, and his book title says it all. The acrimony surrounding divorce usually forces bad decisions, and one simple mistake can end up costing you dearly. Why learn on the job when you can incorporate the experience of thousands of others into your planning. But seriously, if you're going to buy this book (or the one above), you should use the 50 Shades of Grey principle. No-one should ever see you reading it, so get it on your Kindle (and hide your Kindle)!

# Chapter Summary

Audit your situation. Imagine a +/- scale, with zero at the center. To justify continuity, you need to be aiming somewhere in the mid-range on the positive side. Getting there from zero, or maybe just below zero, is viable. However, if you are already further than mid-range on the negative side of the scale, you need to take a serious look at how much effort you are prepared to invest. Just getting back to zero is an unsatisfactory outcome, and will probably not be sufficient to have a dramatic effect on your stress levels.

Visualize how you would like your relationship to be. Then give yourself a reality check; do you have the resources, the knowledge, and the energy to get it there? Or is it simply impossible, or at the very least, highly unlikely? Hope is not a strategy!

In either case, unless you have a better-than-reasonable shot at fixing it, it's time to consider your options.

Budget: can you afford to make the move now, or do you need time to amass a 'war-chest?'

Responsibilities; will you be able to fulfil the essentials from your new situation?

On no account share your plan. Measure your down-side at every step, and bear in mind that 'innocent disclosure' could come back to bite you in the ass.

Keep plans secret and hidden. Seriously. If you make a move, you will discover hidden aspects of your partner's personality that you had never previously encountered.

Don't ever lose sight of your primary objective; to eliminate the stressors which originate from your unsatisfactory, inappropriate, or toxic relationship.

# And Finally

As I said at the beginning, my intention when writing this book was to give you a different perspective on how to deal with Stress, the silent killer. I hope I have succeeded in doing that. The key message I have attempted to deliver is that you do not have to accept your situation, if it is the source of your stress, and in fact you owe it to yourself as a human being to take every possible step to release yourself from the burdens of stress, so that you can excel in your future life.

Whatever you decide to do, equipping yourself with the skills of self-hypnosis will help you relax and focus, the very things that stress obstructs you from doing. If you enjoyed the hypnosis experience, there follows some bonus material which might encourage you to delve deeper into self-hypnosis and find new and different ways to use it for your own personal improvement.

Whatever your choices (and hopefully you now understand that you ALWAYS have choices) I wish you the very best in all your endeavors.

Rick Smith (ricksmith@zonehypnosis.com)

London, England, April 2014.

# Bonus Material:

## Suggestions in Self Hypnosis, And How to Write Them.

If you've followed the instructions, you will have Mastered Self-Hypnosis in a Weekend, which is what we agreed at the start, so well done. You've been superb and you now have a powerful skill which you can develop and polish for the rest of your life, and which will be there for you to call on whenever you feel the need. Mission Accomplished!

And of course if you don't feel like working too hard, and you prefer to use the induction scripts which you downloaded earlier, they are yours to do with what you will!

### Suggestion - The Engine of Hypnotic Change

As we have explored in earlier chapters, the basic objective of hypnosis is to suppress the Critical Faculty (the Conscious Mind) in order to open a direct channel of communication to the Subconscious Mind. Once this is achieved, in the 'trance state', it is then practical to place good-quality behavioural information and instruction directly into the part of the brain which deals with learned behaviour. This is classified as 'Suggestion' and it is the foundation tool of anyone using hypnosis to effect change of any kind.

Professional Hypnosis Practitioners spend around 10% of their training learning how to induce hypnosis in clients, and the other 90% learning the techniques of how to communicate with the client in hypnosis, based largely on Suggestion. This is generally referred to as Therapy, or 'The Work'.

These strategies and techniques vary from the extraordinarily simple (Direct Suggestion) to the immensely complex, and the methods of applying Suggestion can range from 'one-shot' quick-fix techniques to courses of therapy lasting weeks or even months.

## Suggestion and Self-Hypnosis

The differences between Practitioner Induced Hypnotic Therapy and Self-Hypnosis are many and varied. However, the most effective approach for us in this 'teach yourself' context is to keep things as simple as possible. Obviously this limits the volume of information we can include in a suggestion, not only because it heightens the risk of misinterpretation, but also because it is impossible for you to memorize complex scripts and then carry them through the trance induction in order to be able to make the suggestions to yourself, once you are under.

## The Laws of Suggestion

1. Concentrated Attention: Repeated attention to a single idea will inevitably result in its realization.

2. Law of Reverse Effect: The harder you try to do something, the less chance that you will succeed.

3. Law of Dominant Effect: Stronger emotions usually replace weaker ones. Facts have less power than emotions.

Whoever invented these laws gave themselves a Get Out Of Jail Free Card, because it should be obvious to you that not all of these conditions can exist in the same place, at the same time. So the techniques of hypnotic suggestion are loosely based on employing whichever of the 'laws' seem most applicable in any given situation!

## Types of Suggestion

There are a number of different types of suggestion which can be used, such as;

**Direct Suggestion:** The most obvious type of suggestion, which basically says "Feel/Do/Say THIS and you will achieve THAT". Direct suggestion involves a call to action with a motivating goal attached to it. Your subconscious mind receives this type of suggestion and accepts it without resistance, because the suggestion is constructed specifically to tick all the boxes of good advice. Good examples of direct suggestion might be: "You desire those foods which help you to reach your goal" in the case of a dieting suggestion or "You are released from your desire to smoke" in the case of a smoking intervention.

**Indirect Suggestion:** These suggestions usually take the form of a question; however there is never an open-ended answer option. The indirect suggestion offers alternate answers to the question posed, both options having equally beneficial effects. In a Confidence suggestion, you could use something like "Are you gaining confidence because I suggest it or because you are learning to be more confident"? Now you might be mildly contemptuous of the banality of such a suggestion. If someone said that to you in everyday life, you'd find it slightly bizarre. However, remember that in trance you no longer evaluate statements and questions critically, so you would tend to receive such a suggestion without any opinion on the validity of the language used, simply absorbing it as fact. In other words, you would not be puzzled by the use of such simplistic and illogical language whilst in trance.

**Open Ended Suggestion:** This is a way of telling somebody in hypnosis how to feel or act, without giving them any precise position or reason to contradict the suggestion. Again, the subconscious mind will quite happily accept a suggestion such as "You may easily find yourself reflecting on these discoveries you made in trance in the future". Of course, you may not, but that option is virtually eliminated by the open-ended nature of the suggestion.

**Positive Suggestion:** Another foundation stone in our construction of suggestions for Self-Hypnosis will be the use of Positive Suggestion. Simply put, you should generally avoid the use of negative words, such as not, no, never, and so on, because your subconscious mind doesn't like them. Also you might miss a negative word, in which case you could accidentally implant a suggestion completely the opposite of that which was intended. There's a well-known story about a hospital emergency patient whose anesthetic failed whilst in the operating theatre. After the operation, the patient lost the ability to walk, but the surgeons couldn't understand why. In the end, regression hypnotherapy was used to take the patient back and pin point the issue, which turned out to be that he had subconsciously heard the surgeon say "he would never walk again". In actual fact, the surgeon had said "If we hadn't got him to hospital in time, he would never walk again". So the story goes that the misunderstanding was corrected by the hypnotist, and the patient later regained the ability to walk. I have no idea whether this is true, but as a metaphor for positive versus negative suggestion, it is a great illustration of why hypnotic language needs to be clear and unambiguous.

**Negative Suggestions:** Using words like 'no' and 'not' in suggestions can have their benefits. For example, in the hypnotic induction phase, if the hypnotist told you "do not think about the number five" it is probable that you would start to think about the number five. It's a useful tool if you can do it, however for the purpose of Self-Hypnosis we won't be using negative suggestion.

There are numerous other types of suggestion which a Professional Hypnotist might employ, such as Truisms, Bind and Double Bind, Permissive Suggestion and Compounding. However these are not suited to Self-Hypnosis so we'll leave them on one side for now.

You may also have heard about the use of Metaphors, in particular the Ericksonian school of hypnotherapy. This is extraordinarily powerful and effective therapy in the right hands; however it has no practical application in Self-Hypnosis.

## Constructing Suggestions for Self-Hypnosis

At the risk of repetition, it is not practical to take complex scripts with you into the self-hypnotic state, no matter what anyone tells you. Of course you can play recorded scripts to yourself in trance which can be very effective. But for 'pure' Self-Hypnosis, the best approach is to create a simple one-line suggestion which you should be easily able to recall once you have completed the induction phase for yourself. Here are the guidelines;

- Use the Present Tense: Statements of suggestion should be clear that you have achieved your stated objective; "I am a non-smoker" (the use of the negative 'non' in this context is fine because it's more or less a common noun). The future tense is a no-no: "I will be a non-smoker" won't work properly because it's indefinite and opens itself to interpretation by your subconscious, and the obvious question "WHEN will I be a non-smoker?"

- Use the Positive: The realistic possibility that your subconscious could drop a 'not' or 'no' in a suggestion opens you up to the potential to install the exact opposite of what is intended, so steer clear of negative suggestion with Self-Hypnosis. An odd example not to use is "I will not fall asleep whilst driving". Instead you should use "I am awake and alert whilst driving" which eliminates both the negative and the future tense. Remember, simple is good and less is more!
- Don't Use 'Try': The use of 'try' implies the potential to fail. Direct suggestion requires a binary approach, with no latitude for interpretation or excuses.
- Consummate Visualisation: Always visualize something that you are trying to achieve or confirm as if it is already fact, or has already happened.

## S.M.A.R.T. Goal Setting

When you are preparing suggestions for use in Self-Hypnosis, you should focus on structuring your goals according to the following "S.M.A.R.T." acronym, which is as follows:

- **SPECIFIC**: Be precise about what it is you are trying to achieve. A single concept or idea is much easier to shape than a compound set of conditions.
- **MEASURABLE**: This could be a deadline when are going to achieve your Specific Goal, or an amount (of money perhaps) that will satisfy the criteria of 'goal achievement'.

- **ACHIEVABLE**: Here, you need to ensure there are no obstacles which might prevent you from hitting your target.
- **REALISTIC**: Hypnosis is an enabler. It is not a miracle worker, so make sure you are setting out to do something reasonable, not overstretching yourself beyond what is realistic.
- **TIMELY**: Your plan should have a timetable which you know is achievable. If you are too aggressive with your deadline, no amount of hypnotic empowerment is going to get you there.

## Using the Suggestion Phrase

If you are going to use Suggestion in Self-Hypnosis, just follow the simple steps below;

Prepare your environment, exactly as you did in the earlier exercises. Calmly run thorough your plan (either out-loud or internally), like this:

- In a moment, I am going to breathe in, and when I breathe out, I will take myself down into hypnosis, as I have often done before.
- I will take as much time as I need to become completely relaxed and ready to work on my (whatever you are planning to do)
- In my relaxed hypnotic state, I will suggest to myself: (insert your one-line suggestion 'script' 'x')
- I will take my time to thoroughly process my suggestion about 'x'

- When I am done, I will emerge myself to my full waking state, feeling great and ready to incorporate my new learning/behaviour/plan into my life.

When you are ready, do it!

## Writing Your Self-Suggestion

Following the rules and guidelines above, you should be able to construct a one-line suggestion script for just about anything.

Once you are in trance, and you can repeat your suggestion, you will release your full imagination which will develop the imagery or sensory experience of achieving your objective. It is a good idea to have completed the 'SMART' exercise earlier in the section, so that you have a 'model' of what you want to see, and how you want to feel.

The Suggestion that you construct is the trigger to make all this happen, so you should make it as precise and unambiguous as you can manage. Here are some examples:

"As the days and weeks go by I am...."

- Paying more attention to the healthy food I eat.
- Enjoying the freedom of living without fizzy drinks.
- Growing more relaxed and contended in myself.
- Easily able to manage the energetic requirements of my career.
- Filled with love and appreciation for my family/friends/etc.

- Excited to discover what the future holds for me as I reach my potential in every way.

I'm sure you get the drift by now, and you can easily construct appropriate suggestions for yourself, to suit your personal Self-Hypnosis objectives.

## And Remember

Always accept the hypnotic experience as it comes to you. Avoid asking yourself questions such as "am I hypnotized?" and simply get on with the process as explained above. Remember that you are putting aside your critical faculty in order to make full use of your powerful subconscious mind. The more questions you ask, the more you continue to engage your critical faculty, which will block your progress. The harder you try, the tougher it will be to succeed, so simply relax and let the hypnosis work in its own way. Practice makes perfect. It is not the subjective experience that matters, it is the outcome. Trust yourself and the process and it WILL work for you.

# Other Books by Rick Smith

E-Cig Revolution; How to Save a Million Lives and a Billion Healthcare Dollars

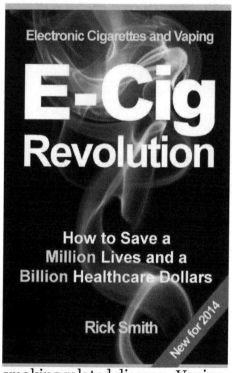

Find out all about the FIRST REAL ALTERNATIVE to smoking cigarettes.Electronic Cigarettes and Vaping provides the first real alternative to smoking tobacco. So how does it work, and why should you consider it?

Smokers die, on average, nine years earlier than non-smokers. Over 8m Americans live with smoking related disease. Vaping eliminates the harmful carcinogenic chemicals present in tobacco smoke. E-cigarettes cost a fraction of the price of normal cigarettes.

But there's a Covert Conspiracy that threatens to BAN THEM COMPLETELY. In E-Cig Revolution, you'll discover a scandalous global war being fought out between Government, Regulators, Health, and Industry for control of the lucrative E-Cigarette industry: Why is the Healthcare Industry terrified to declare E-Cigs to be safe? Who's funding Governments and Regulators to block access to E-Cigs? And what about the stand-off between Big Pharma and Big Tobacco, and who will ultimately triumph? How the shelves could be cleared for years to come if the wrong people get their way!

You'll get the latest information on how to switch, what to buy, and what to expect. There's a bewildering array of competing products out there, all claiming to be the best. How do you decide what's right for you? What's the closest thing to 'real' smoking, so you won't slip back into cigarettes? Should you go disposable or rechargeable, shop-bought or online? What about nicotine strengths and different flavors? How to switch; step-by-step or all in one go?

In fact, everything you need to make the right decision, quit smoking, and break free of your tobacco addiction. Then decide for yourself: Live Well or Die Young? If you've tried to quit smoking and failed, with patches, gum, hypnosis or acupuncture, E-Cigarettes could be the lifeline you've been searching for. Get your health back: clearer breathing, whiter teeth, fresher breath, and more energy! Save up to 90% over the cost of smoking cigarettes! That's thousands every year! No more standing outside in the rain and the cold to get your nicotine fix! Free yourself today, and live a longer, healthier, and happier life!

The E-Cig revolution will change your life, the lives of

your family and kids, and could be the biggest boost to public health since the eradication of smallpox, tuberculosis and plague! Join the Revolution; you truly have Nothing to Lose and Everything to Gain!

How to Master Self-Hypnosis in a Weekend – The Simple, Systematic and Successful Way to Get Everything You Want.

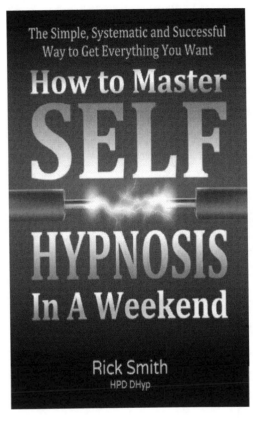

Hundreds of books have been published about Self-Hypnosis, so what makes this one special? Well, maybe you're trying Self-Hypnosis for the first time, or maybe you've tried before and failed. Whatever the case, you're looking for results, otherwise you'll probably waste a lot of time, and come away disappointed and disillusioned. You need a System.

In 'How to Master Self-Hypnosis in a Weekend' British Hypnotist Rick Smith demonstrates a step-by-step system which anyone can use to succeed. Everything you need, included freely downloadable script recordings, is provided. Using this book, you will quickly master the key Self-Hypnosis techniques that will enable you to drop easily and quickly into a comfortable trance anywhere, anytime.

You'll also learn how to use your new Self-Hypnosis skills for relaxation and recreation, how to use Self-Hypnosis to control stress and to center yourself professionally, how to attack bad habits, such as smoking, drinking, over-eating, in fact anything that you feel the need to change, and how to empower yourself for motivation, focus and commitment. You'll also discover how to avoid the common mistakes that other people make; they don't practice often enough, so they fail to master the key techniques; they don't get the 'set-up' right, so they become distracted; they cling on to their inhibitions, so they never release their restrictive self-control; and they try to analyse too much, rather than allowing nature do its best work.

If you follow these step-by-step instructions you will quickly learn everything you need to know in order to master the simple skills of Self-Hypnosis. With regular use, you will acquire a powerful secret weapon that will serve you in almost any aspect of your life. And the more you do it, the better you will become. It's easy, it's quick, and it's really fun to do!

50920332R00085

Made in the USA
San Bernardino, CA
08 July 2017